Ethical Dilemmas in Allied Health

Second Edition

Janine M. Idziak, Ph.D.
Loras College

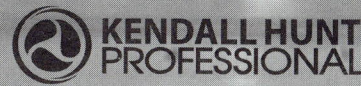

Cover image © Dmitry Kushch, 2009
Used under License from Shutterstock, Inc

Copyright © 2000 by Simon & Kolz Publishing, LLC.

Copyright © 2010 by Kendall Hunt Publishing Company

ISBN 978-0-7575-6371-3

All rights reserved. No part of this publication may be reproduced, stored in a retrieval system, or transmitted, in any form or by any means, electronic, mechanical, photocopying, recording, or otherwise, without the prior written permission of the copyright owner.

Printed in the United States of America
10 9 8 7 6 5 4 3 2 1

For Carol Reffner

Contents

	Preface	vii
Chapter 1	Ethics for Health Care	1
Chapter 2	Ethics Committees: A Resource for Resolving Ethical Dilemmas	25

Part One	**Ethical Issues at the Beginning of Life**	**29**
Chapter 3	The Abortion Debate	31
Chapter 4	Assisted Reproductive Technologies	49
Chapter 5	Treatment Decisions for Seriously Ill Newborns	65

Part Two	**Ethical Issues at the End of Life**	**79**
Chapter 6	Making Decisions about Using or Forgoing Life-Sustaining Treatments	81
Chapter 7	Proxy Decision Making and Advance Directives	97
Chapter 8	The Dilemma of Assisted Nutrition and Hydration	113
Chapter 9	Treatment Decisions for Vegetative State Patients	131
Chapter 10	Euthanasia and Assisted Suicide	147

Part Three	**Issues of Professionalism**	**165**
Chapter 11	Confidentiality	167
Chapter 12	Workplace Ethics	177
Chapter 13	Ethical and Religious Objections to Health Care Practices	191
Chapter 14	Multicultural Perspectives in Health Care	203

Part Four	**Special Topics**	**215**
Chapter 15	Research and Experimentation Involving Human Subjects	217
Chapter 16	Stem Cell Research	233
Chapter 17	Issues in Organ Procurement and Allocation	243
Chapter 18	Genetics in the 21st Century: The DNA Frontier	259
	Index	273

Preface

Over the past several decades, health care ethics has developed and flourished as an academic discipline. The field now includes a standard set of topics. Issues such as abortion, assisted reproduction, terminating life-sustaining treatment, euthanasia and assisted suicide, confidentiality, and the allocation of scarce medical resources are commonly covered in textbooks on health care ethics. However, the perspective assumed in these textbooks may be limited in comparison with the actual range of health care services and types of health care professionals. Case studies on ethical dilemmas typically focus on physicians and nurses in a hospital setting.

This textbook, on the other hand, approaches the standard problems of health care ethics *from the perspective of the allied health fields*. Case studies always involve allied health professionals, giving recognition to them as an integral part of the care giving team.

Health care is no longer synonymous with the hospital setting, but includes assisted living complexes, long-term care facilities, home health care services, and hospice facilities. This book is broader in scope than many textbooks in health care ethics in including examples beyond the acute care setting.

Many health care facilities have established ethics committees to help patients, family members, and health care providers work through difficult ethical dilemmas. This textbook recognizes the increasing role ethics committees are playing in health care. It refers to the use of ethics committees and includes exercises that invite students to assume the roles of ethics committee members.

Apart from the first and second background chapters, each chapter in the book has the same structure. The introductory section lists the issues to be considered in the chapter. The chapter includes one or more case studies describing concrete situations in which these issues arise, with expository sections discussing the issues. At the end of the chapter is a summary section listing key terms and concepts used in the chapter and the key points made about the issues discussed. Finally, there is a section entitled "For Further Discussion" which asks students to think critically about the material in the chapter and to apply principles they have learned to concrete cases. They are also asked to role play discussion of ethical dilemmas and to relate issues to their personal experiences. In sum, the section "For Further Discussion" invites students to become active participants in "doing ethics."

Although the case studies presented are hypothetical, they are based on particular cases or types of cases that actually occur. The case studies are generally written as if they are currently taking place. This has been done deliberately to simulate the actual ethical decision making process. When we have to make a tough ethical decision, we often do not know exactly what the outcome will be. This is part of the challenge of "doing ethics."

This textbook may be used at either the undergraduate or graduate level. Supplementary ethical, religious, and legal materials have been made available and may be selected to enrich the basic printed text. The text may be used in its entirety in a course devoted specifically to ethics, or selected chapters may be used in conjunction with other courses in allied health. If the text is individualized by an instructor in this way, the selection should always include the first chapter on ethical theory and the second chapter on ethics committees.

Web Resources

Resources for both students and instructors are available at the Kendall Hunt Professional web site located at http://www.edah2.com. There you will find online teaching tools, additional Internet, print, and audiovisual resources, a guide for doing research in bioethics, and JCAHCO guidelines.

Acknowledgments

As a professor of philosophy, my academic work in the field of bioethics has been greatly enriched by the "hands on" experience afforded me by serving on ethics committees at various health care facilities. In particular, I want to extend my thanks to Mercy Medical Center and Stonehill Franciscan Services in Dubuque, Iowa.

My work as chair of the Medical-Moral Commission of the Archdiocese of Dubuque in preparing a handbook on health care ethics provided the occasion for extensive searches of the literature on bioethics. I have drawn on some of this work in preparing this textbook.

Finally, I am grateful to Loras College for granting me released time from teaching to pursue work in the field of bioethics.

Janine Marie Idziak, Ph.D.
Dubuque, Iowa
May 2009

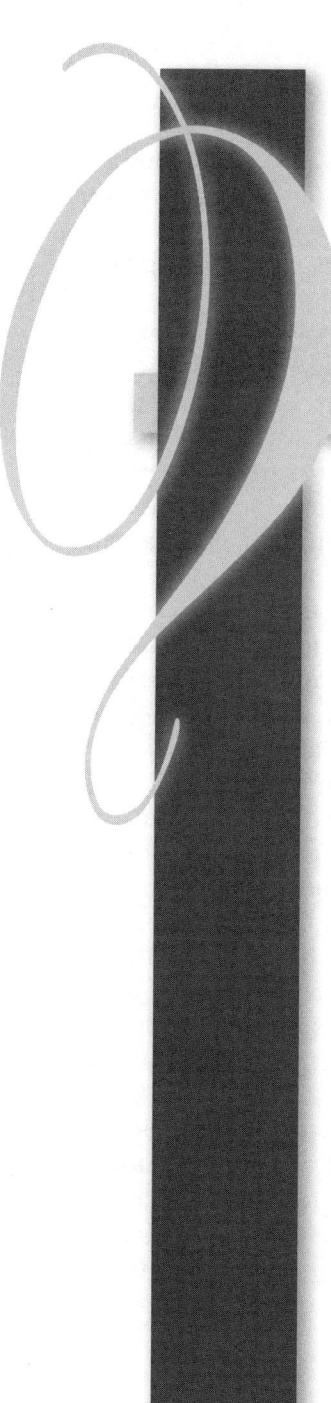

Chapter 1

Ethics for Health Care

What Is Ethics?

Ethics asks us to stand back and evaluate our actions. It asks us to judge that some actions ought to be done and that others ought to be avoided.

In the minds of some, ethics consists in nothing but a set of rules governing behavior—rules that have often been superimposed by other people. Ethics is thought of as nothing more than a list of "do's" and "don'ts."

However, contemporary philosophers have presented ethics as an enterprise fostering human happiness and fulfillment. On this view, *the purpose of ethical reflection is to consider the choices and courses of action that most promote the fulfillment of persons and the community.* (1) Understood in this way, "doing ethics" is a very positive activity.

The Ethical Dimensions of Health Care

Decision making in health care often involves more than just the brute medical facts of the case. Ethical principles and values will be the determining factor in which course of action is chosen.

By way of example, consider decisions arising from the use of fertility drugs. Fertility drugs can result in multifetal pregnancies; that is, pregnancies where more than one fetus is conceived and carried. A famous case is that of septuplets born to the McCaugheys in Carlisle, Iowa. (2) It is a medical fact that multifetal pregnancies, "particularly those which involve more than triplets, can cause health risks for the mother such as an increased risk for hypertension, gestational diabetes, anemia, as well as the side effects from tocolytic agents often used to stop premature contractions." (2) Another medical fact is that multifetal pregnancies are risky for the babies themselves. Multifetal pregnancies frequently end in miscarriage or stillbirth, and the risk increases with the number of fetuses. (3) Moreover, even when they do survive, such babies are nearly always born prematurely, with all the complications prematurity entails. Thus "multiple babies have 12 times as great a chance of dying in infancy," and "if they survive, they face all sorts of potential problems later in life, from cerebral palsy to kidney and bowel problems to blindness to mental retardation." (3)

Because of the risks to the babies themselves involved in a multifetal pregnancy, the option of "selective reduction" may be recommended. In selective reduction, several fetuses are aborted so that the remaining fetuses stand a better chance of being born healthy. (3) Whether this option is chosen will depend on the couple's views about the moral permissibility of abortion. Everyone involved could agree on the medical facts of the case—the risks involved in a multifetal pregnancy. However, one couple may choose selective reduction while another couple (like the McCaugheys) may reject it because of their different views on the ethical permissibility of abortion. Their respective *ethical* views ultimately determine which course of action is taken *medically*.

Many health care facilities now have ethics committees in place. (See chapter 2.) Many large health care systems employ professional ethicists to address ethical issues on a full-time basis. Just as it is common practice to consult with specialists about medical care, so ethics consultation services are now being offered to help patients, families, and health care providers work through difficult ethical dilemmas. (See chapter 2.) Thus ethics has very much become a part of contemporary health care services.

Health care professionals should study ethics so that they can be sensitive to the ethical principles and values that enter into the decision-making processes of patients and their families. The study of ethics will likewise help prepare them to meet ethics standards set for health care facilities and by their own professional associations. Finally, studying ethics will enable health care professionals to participate fully in the ethics services offered by the facilities and agencies that employ them.

Two Levels of Ethical Inquiry in Health Care

Ethical issues concerning health care can arise at different levels. Obviously, ethical questions can arise *in the care of individual patients.* Should 80-year-old John, who has Alzheimer's disease, be resuscitated if he suffers a cardiac arrest? Should he be given antibiotics if he develops pneumonia? Eleanor has been unconscious for a year, and physicians think it very unlikely that she will ever regain consciousness. Should her tube feeding be discontinued so that she can be allowed to die? Should Jackie abort a much wanted child because prenatal diagnosis shows that her fetus has a genetic disorder? These types of questions belong to the category of *clinical ethics.*

At the same time, ethical questions can arise about *how a health care facility or service is operated.* For example, ethical questions can be raised about the financing of health care. Is it right for a physician who is part of a health maintenance organization (HMO) to refrain from prescribing a particular drug for a patient because the drug is too costly? Or, how much "charity care" should the local community hospital provide to patients who have lost their jobs and, along with it, their health insurance? Ethical questions can also arise regarding a health care facility's treatment of its employees. Is it appropriate for a hospital to discourage unionization on the part of its employees? Was the last merit raise for employees fairly handled? Should a married health care worker with children be dismissed if she refuses to come to work during an epidemic of an infectious disease? Yet another concern today is how the ethical value of confidentiality can be preserved with the computerization of medical records. All of these questions belong to the realm of *organizational ethics.*

While this textbook will give primary attention to issues in clinical ethics, some issues from the realm of organizational ethics will also be addressed.

Ethical Theories

An ethical theory is a way of organizing our ethical reflection and deliberations. It directs us to the features of a situation that are relevant to making a determination of rightness or wrongness of action.

Various ethical theories have been brought to bear on issues in health care ethics. For each theory, we describe its standard for determining rightness and wrongness of action, give an example of how the theory applies to a particular issue in health care, and discuss the plausibility of the theory as a whole.

Principalism

In *Principles of Biomedical Ethics,* a book that has now become a classic of contemporary health care ethics, Tom Beauchamp and James Childress reduce all of health care ethics to four basic principles: *autonomy, nonmaleficence, beneficence,* and *justice.* (4) These principles are sometimes referred to as the "Georgetown mantra" because of the association of the philosophers who developed them with the Kennedy Institute of Ethics at Georgetown University. (4, 5)

The word "autonomy" is of Greek derivation, and "originally referred to the self-rule or self-governance of independent city-states." (4) By extension, autonomy refers to self-determination by an individual of the course of his or her own life:

> Personal autonomy is, at a minimum, self-rule that is free from both controlling interference by others and from limitations, such as inadequate understanding, that prevent meaningful choice. The autonomous individual acts freely in accordance with a self-chosen plan, analogous to the way an independent government manages its territories and sets its policies. (4)

Respecting an individual's autonomy entails acknowledging "that person's right to hold views, to make choices, and to take actions based on personal values and beliefs." (4) In the context of health care, respecting autonomy means involving the patient in decisions about medical treatment, and allowing the individual to make the final decision in these matters. It also means giving the patient reasonable control and choice when interacting with the health care system in general. The principle of autonomy is related to Kantian ethics (see below) in that violating a person's autonomy "is to treat that person merely as a means, that is, in accordance with others' goals without regard to that person's own goals." (4)

The principle of nonmaleficence "asserts an obligation not to inflict harm on others." (4) In a health care context, it is associated with the maxim *primum non nocere;* that is, "above all [or first] do not harm." (4) Nonmaleficence includes "not imposing *risks* of harm," and is related to the concepts of negligence and the standard of due care. (4) Beneficence has to do with contributing to the welfare of other people, so that the principle of beneficence refers to a moral obligation to act for the benefit of others. This principle is related to nonmaleficence in that "no sharp break exists on the continuum from not inflicting harm to providing benefit." (4) However, the principle of beneficence potentially demands more than the principle of nonmaleficence "because agents must take positive steps to help others, not merely refrain from harmful acts." (4)

On an intuitive level, justice concerns "fair, equitable, and appropriate treatment in light of what is due or owed to persons." (4) Talk of justice often refers specifically to the concept of distributive justice, which "concerns the distribution of such social benefits and burdens as medical services, welfare payments, public offices, taxes, and military service." (6) Attempts have been made to articulate more specific principles governing the distribution of social benefits and burdens. These attempts include the principle of equality, the principle of need, the principle of contribution, and the principle of effort. (6; see also 4)

The principle of equality, as the name indicates, embodies a radical egalitarianism. Everyone is to be treated the same in all respects, and all social benefits and burdens are to be distributed equally. Everyone, so to speak, is entitled to the same slice of the pie, and everyone must bear an equal part of the social load. The principle of need is an extension of the egalitarian principle. (6) According to the principle of need, goods should be parceled out according to individual need so that those who have greater needs receive a greater share. The outcome will be one of equality, however, for given the fact that everyone's needs will be met, everyone will end up at the same level. The treatment of individuals will be equal although the proportion of goods they receive will be different. (6)

The principle of contribution, on the other hand, maintains that "everyone should get back that proportion of social goods that is the result of his or her productive labor." (6) To use an everyday example, this principle holds that "if two people work to grow potatoes and the first works twice as long or twice as hard as the second, then the first should be entitled to twice as large a share of the harvest." (6)

Finally, the principle of effort asserts that "the degree of effort made by the individual should determine the proportion of goods received by the individual." (6) Again using an everyday example, this principle holds that "the file clerk who works just as hard as the president of a company should receive the same proportion of social goods as the president" while "those who are lazy and refuse to exert themselves will receive proportionally less than those who work hard." (6) This principle is attractive in seeming to capture "our sense of what is fair—that those who do their best should be similarly rewarded, while those who do less than their best should be less well rewarded." (6)

Ethicists acknowledge that a comprehensive theory of justice may include more than one (or possibly all) of these more specific principles of distributive justice. (4, 6) Indeed, it has been claimed that, as a matter of fact, "most societies invoke several of these material principles in framing public policies, appealing to different principles in different spheres and contexts." (4)

According to the principalist theory, ethical dilemmas are generated when more than one of the basic principles (autonomy, nonmaleficence, beneficence, and justice) are applicable to a situation and the principles conflict in directing what course of action ought to be taken. For example, a patient who is dying may say that she wants "everything done," including care in the intensive care unit (ICU). On the other hand, her physician may believe that ICU care would be futile in prolonging her life and might take a bed away from an emergency case coming into the hospital whose recovery would be greatly helped by ICU care. This case involves a conflict between patient autonomy and justice in the allocation of health care resources. Autonomy directs that the patient should be placed in the ICU unit. Justice, on the other hand, and more specifically, the principle of need, argues against this. The patient in an emergency situation can benefit from ICU care in a way that the terminally ill patient in question cannot, and thus can claim a greater need for ICU care. In such cases of conflict, a judgment must be made as to which principle (autonomy or justice) is weightier and should take precedence in that particular situation. (4) One drawback of this scheme of doing ethics is the difficulty of making such determinations in a non-arbitrary way.

As will be seen throughout this text, the principle of autonomy has come to occupy a central place in contemporary health care ethics and practice. For example, it provides an ethical grounding for the development of advance directives. (See chapter 7.) Moreover, it is now standard practice that patients give their "informed consent" to medical treatments and procedures and to various practices within a health care institution and, "since the mid-1970's, the primary justification advanced for requirements of informed consent has been to protect autonomous choice." (4) Or again, the HIPAA (Health Insurance Portability and Accountability Act) Privacy Rule imposes stringent administrative requirements on the collection, maintenance, transmission, use, and disclosure of individually identifiable health information. (7) According to the U.S. Office for Civil Rights, the Privacy Rule "gives patients more control over their health information" and enables them "to make informed choices when seeking care and reimbursement for care based on how personal health information may be used." (8) From this perspective, the HIPAA privacy regulations are in line with the ethical emphasis on individual autonomy.

The emphasis currently being placed on patient autonomy is, at least in part, a reaction to the paternalistic way in which the health care professions were practiced at one time. The health care providers were the ones who made the treatment decisions, and the patient and family members tended to go along with what they said without raising questions. The emphasis on patient autonomy may also reflect the American emphasis on individualism. (5, 9)

While no one is advocating a return to a purely paternalist approach on the part of health care providers, some concern is now being raised that the pendulum has swung too far in the other direction. There is concern that patient autonomy has gone too far and that some limits on it are in order. For example, some are arguing that a patient should not be entitled to receive medical treatments that are futile and that health care providers have the right to override patient wishes when futile treatments are wanted. (See chapter 6.) Others offer a more radical criticism of the very concept of patient autonomy, maintaining that a focus on the patient alone is misguided. (5)

Out of feminist work in ethics has come the *ethics of care*. This approach to ethics is described in the following way:

> . . . girls, being brought up by mothers, identify with them, while males must define themselves through separation from their mothers. . . . Thus while masculinity is defined by separation and threatened by intimacy, femininity is defined through attachment and threatened by separation; girls come to understand themselves as imbedded within a network of personal relationships. . . .
>
> The feminine voice in ethics attends to the particular other, thinks in terms of responsibilities to care for others, is sensitive to our interconnectedness, and strives to preserve relationships. It contrasts with the masculine voice, which speaks in terms of justice and rights, stresses consistency and principles, and emphasizes the autonomy of the individual and impartiality in one's dealings with others. (10)

This feminist approach to ethics is "frequently described in terms of webs or networks" (5) and emphasizes "relationships and connections" rather than "isolated individuals." (5)

It has been claimed that the ethics of care is already part of the way we naturally reason in health care ethics:

> Looking at ethics committees, Sichel argues that a feminist ethics of caring is often part of the ethics committee's deliberations. She uses as an

example the case of an incompetent elderly patient whose wishes are known but whose children disagree about what course to follow. She accurately notes that, although the committee will support following the patient's wishes, it will go to considerable lengths and spend considerable time in an attempt to obtain consensus about this course from all the children, believing that it has a duty to care about the family as well as the patient. It would appear that if the patient's wishes were the only important factor, the course of action desired by the patient should be followed immediately, rather than after the children have been persuaded to agree. (5)

In sum, rather than focusing exclusively on what the patient wants (the principle of patient autonomy), the ethics of care directs us to take into account all the players in an ethical dilemma.

Consequentialist Theories

Consequentialist ethical theories, as the name indicates, judge rightness and wrongness of action on the basis of the consequences of action. The right action to perform is the one which, among the alternatives, has the best consequences overall. Or, if all the possible courses of action have negative consequences overall, the right action to perform is the one with the least bad consequences. Different consequentialist theories are generated by the range of consequences taken into account. An *ethical egoist* considers the consequences only for himself or herself as the agent of the action. The more popular (and plausible) theory of *utilitarianism* considers the consequences for everyone to be affected by the action, taking into account the impact on other people as well as the agent of the action. (11)

Historically, utilitarianism was formulated by two British philosophers, Jeremy Bentham (12) and John Stuart Mill (13), in the eighteenth and nineteenth centuries. It is commonly known as the philosophy of "the greatest good for the greatest number." (14) To better understand this system of ethics, let us consider how it would approach a particular ethical issue.

Consider reasons offered for and against surrogate motherhood, where a woman is artificially inseminated to produce and carry to term a child for a contracting couple. On the one hand, surrogacy provides a much wanted child to an infertile couple. It allows the child to be biologically related to the father. And, given the shortage of children available for adoption, it can provide an infertile couple with a child more quickly. On the other hand, the surrogate mother can become attached to the child she is carrying and find giving up the child to be emotionally traumatic. Indeed, she may decide she wants to keep the child, with ensuing court battles. If the surrogate is willing to give up the child but is herself married and has her own children, these children may experience a sense of loss at being deprived of a sibling. If the child born in a surrogacy arrangement turns out to be mentally or physically handicapped, neither the surrogate mother nor the contracting couple may want the child, and the child may end up in a state institution. (15, 16, 17)

When analyzed, all these reasons for and against surrogacy represent positive and negative consequences of surrogate motherhood. Consequences are discussed for a variety of people impacted by the surrogate motherhood arrangement: the infertile couple, the woman who serves as a surrogate mother, children of the surrogate mother, the child born through the surrogacy arrangement, and society at large. Thus the above paragraph represents a utilitarian way of thinking about the ethical permissibility of surrogate motherhood.

Since the time of Bentham and Mill, several different types of utilitarianism have been formulated. Perhaps the simplest form of utilitarianism is *act-utilitarian,* which focuses on particular courses of action. (11) What would be the consequences of allowing a hypothetical John Taylor to commit assisted suicide when he is terminally ill and in severe pain and requests it? Other types of utilitarianism, rather than focusing on particular actions, consider the consequences of adopting a certain set of rules (11), or the consequences of people generally performing a certain type of action. (18) In other words, what would be the consequences of adopting a state law (a rule) which allows assisted suicide? Or what would be the consequences of most people who are terminally ill and in severe pain committing assisted suicide? Some versions of utilitarianism (such as that first formulated by Bentham and Mill) judge consequences hedonistically, in terms of the pleasure and pain produced. (12, 13) On the other hand, a recent variant of utilitarianism makes such judgments in terms of people's actual preferences. (19)

For the utilitarian, no action is intrinsically right or wrong. Rightness and wrongness are determined entirely by consequences. Consider, for example, the issue of confidentiality. According to the utilitarian, "if violating confidentiality seems necessary to produce a state of affairs in which happiness is increased, then the violation is justified." (20) This might occur, for instance, when "someone's life is in danger or someone is being tried for a serious crime and the testimony of a physician is needed to help establish her innocence." (20)

Utilitarianism requires us to consider consequences of actions not only for ourselves, but for everyone who will be affected by what we do. In this regard, John Stuart Mill commended utilitarianism on religious grounds:

> . . . the happiness which forms the utilitarian standard of what is right in conduct is not the agent's own happiness but that of all concerned. As between his own happiness and that of others, utilitarianism requires him to be as strictly impartial as a disinterested and benevolent spectator. In the golden rule of Jesus of Nazareth, we read the complete spirit of the ethics of utility. "To do as you would be done by," and "to love your neighbor as yourself," constitute the ideal perfection of utilitarian morality. (13)

As another point in favor of the theory, a utilitarian might point to the extent to which we ordinarily look at consequences of action in deciding what we ought to do. In other words, it might be argued that utilitarianism reflects our ordinary ethical thinking. In addition, some are attracted to utilitarianism because it forces us to take time to figure out and consider the consequences of our actions. Utilitarianism forces us to be reflective about ethical decisions rather than making them quickly on the basis of initial reactions.

On the other hand, there are some practical difficulties with applying utilitarianism. Do we always have the time to consider all possible consequences of our actions before a choice must be made? Consider the case of an emergency room physician who has to decide whether to use a new drug on a patient brought in with a heart attack. Or again, can we really determine what all the consequences of our actions may be in the long run? Our actions can have unforeseeable ripple effects. (21) For example, marriage partners often meet in college settings. The partner a person selects will determine much about the course of that person's life; for example, number of children, the particular children he or she has, home environment, geographical mobility, levels of personal satisfaction and happiness. But can anyone foresee these possible consequences when choosing which college to attend?

Another objection to utilitarianism is an intuitive feeling that factors other than consequences do count in making moral judgments. For example, the very fact that a promise has been made should count for something, apart from the consequences of keeping or breaking the promise. (22) Or we believe that it is simply unjust to punish an innocent person, even if punishing him in the circumstances might have good consequences overall. (23) A final and very important criticism of utilitarianism will be discussed in the framework of Kantian ethics.

Kant's Categorical Imperative

An ethical theory that makes moral judgments on the basis of considerations other than the consequences of actions is that of the eighteenth century German philosopher Immanuel Kant. Kant named his fundamental ethical principle the *categorical imperative*. He gave different formulations of the categorical imperative, stating his fundamental ethical principle in different ways. The two most famous formulations are the *universal law* formula, and the *end in itself* formula. It is the end in itself formula of the categorical imperative that has recently been used in dealing with issues in health care ethics.

Kant stated the end in itself formula in this way: "So act as to treat humanity, whether in thine own person or in that of any other, in every case as an end withal, never as a means only...." (24) This is an explanation of what he means:

> According to this formulation, rational creatures should always treat other rational creatures as ends in themselves and never as only means to ends. This formulation underscores Kant's belief that every human being has an inherent worth resulting from the sheer possession of rationality. We must always act in a way that respects this humanity in others and in ourselves. (11)

According to Kant, we act wrongly if we merely "use" another person to get something we want. We act rightly only if we treat human beings, both other people and ourselves, as beings having inherent, intrinsic worth. Kant's end in itself formula is sometimes referred to as a principle of "respect for persons." (17)

For example, some of the arguments offered against the ethical permissibility of surrogate motherhood are applications of this Kantian moral principle:

> This makes it appear that surrogacy is unethical because of the type of practice it is, namely, a form of exploitation. According to one writer: "When a woman provides womb service, the feminist issue surfaces. Women object to being baby factories or sex objects because it offends their human dignity." And further: "This is going to end up as the final exploitation of women. It is always going to be poor women who have the babies and rich women who get them."
>
> ... to treat one's body as a mere means to the ends of others is degrading. It could be viewed as a violation of Kant's supreme moral principle, the categorical imperative, which prohibits treating persons merely as a means. (25)

Both utilitarians and Kantians have arguments pertaining to surrogate motherhood, but their arguments are of different types.

It is very important to recognize that utilitarians and Kantians can come to different conclusions about the right thing to do in a particular case. Suppose, for example, that a teenage girl is dying of cancer and that all known treatments have failed to help her. Her physicians suggest use of an experimental drug. The physicians do not believe that the drug will help this girl. In fact, they candidly tell her parents that she is likely to suffer from fever and vomiting if she takes it (which will increase her suffering as she dies). However, if she does take the drug, the physicians will gain information about how cancer patients tolerate it. This information will be valuable in using the drug in the future with other cancer patients who may be helped by it. (26) A Kantian would be against giving the girl the experimental drug because she would simply be used to gain knowledge for the benefit of other people. A utilitarian, on the other hand, would favor the administration of the experimental drug because of the good consequences overall. While the girl will suffer, the negative value of her suffering will be outweighed by the good consequences for other people.

This case illustrates another objection brought against utilitarianism; namely, that it can justify sacrificing the individual for the sake of the group. (21) On the other hand, Kant's end in itself formula of the categorical imperative has been criticized on the grounds that "it is not always clear when people are being treated as ends and when as means." (11) For example, Kant judged prostitution to be immoral "because, by selling their sexual services, prostitutes allow themselves to be treated as means." (11) However, there is a sense in which anyone who works for a wage also sells his or her services. (11) So "does that mean that we are all being treated immorally, because our employers are presumably hiring us as a means to advance their own ends?" (11) This question might be answered negatively on the grounds that we have freely agreed to do the work. But then the same is true of the prostitute (11) so that the counter-point does not hold up.

Rights, Duties, and Obligations

Talk about "rights" we have is very much a part of the language of ethical discourse. As one ethicist has commented:

> Statements of rights provide vital protections of life, liberty, expression, and property. They protect against oppression, unequal treatment, intolerance, arbitrary invasion of privacy, and the like. Some philosophers and framers of political declarations even regard rights as the basic language for expressing the moral point of view. (4)

A *right* may be defined as a justified claim that individuals and groups can make upon other individuals or upon society. In other words, "to have a right is to be in a position to determine, by one's choices, what others should do or need not do." (4)

A focus on rights is related to a particular conception of the nature and purpose of ethics that sees its function as protecting the interests of individuals. Hence, if rights "are our primary instruments to this end, then moral action-guides are rights-based." (4) Even if one does not accept a rights-based account of ethics as a comprehensive and complete ethical theory, at least one can see rights as "a statement of certain minimal and enforceable rules that communities and individuals must observe in their treatment of all persons." (4)

Rights are grounded in and justified by our ethical principles and rules. For example, we speak of a "right to privacy." Basically, this is a person's right to control access to himself or herself. This right includes limited access to information about the person and to bodily products and objects intimately associated with the person. It also extends to unwanted interventions in zones of secrecy, anonymity, seclusion or solitude, and encompasses limited access to the person's intimate relationships with friends, lovers, spouses, physicians, and the like. (4) One justification for asserting a right to privacy lies in the ethical theory of principalism and its principle of autonomy. Specifically, "we often respect persons by respecting their autonomous wishes not to be observed, touched, or intruded upon." (4) Or again, the notion of a "right to health care" has surfaced. This can again be related to principalism; more exactly, to the principle of distributive justice, and the application of this principle to the allocation of health care resources. (4)

Another dimension of our ethical discourse is talk about "duties," or interchangeably, about "obligations." (27) The twentieth century English philosopher W.D. Ross formulated an entire ethical theory based on the concept of duty. (4, 22, 27, 28) Ross spoke of *prima facie* duties; that is, of duties "at first sight" or "other things being equal." (28) In other words, a prima facie duty "dictates what I should do when other relevant factors in a situation are not considered." (28) Ross claimed that the following prima facie duties are generally recognized on an intuitive basis:

1. Duties of fidelity: telling the truth, keeping promises.
2. Duties of reparation: righting the wrongs we have done to others.
3. Duties of gratitude: recognizing the services others have done for us.
4. Duties of justice: preventing a distribution of pleasure or happiness that is not in keeping with the merit of the people involved.
5. Duties of beneficence: helping to better the condition of other beings with respect to virtue, intelligence, or pleasure.

6. Duties of self-improvement: bettering ourselves with respect to virtue or intelligence.
7. Duties of nonmaleficence: avoiding or preventing an injury to others. (28)

Ross makes a distinction between prima facie duties and our *actual duty* in a particular situation. In some cases, several prima facie duties may apply and be in conflict in what they tell us to do. This is reminiscent of what can happen with the theory of principalism described above. Ross offers two guidelines for determining our actual duty in such cases. First, in the case of two conflicting prima facie duties, he maintains that one's actual duty consists in the act that is in accord with the more stringent prima facie obligation. Further, when several prima facie duties are in conflict, he holds that one's actual duty is the act that has the greatest balance of prima facie rightness over prima facie wrongness. However, a weakness in Ross's theory is that he does not give us any concrete directions for determining when one duty is "more stringent" than another or for determining the "balance" of prima facie rightness over wrongness. (28)

In spite of this weakness, it has been observed that Ross's theory is useful in a health care context in encouraging "each person responsible for patient care to reflect on the prima facie obligations that he or she has toward those people and to set aside one of those obligations only when morally certain that another obligation takes precedence." (28)

Natural Law

The idea of a natural law goes back to Greek and Roman legal thought, where one finds this idea among Stoics and in the writings of Cicero. Natural law theory flourished in the high and late Middle Ages. In this period, the classic statement of natural law theory was given by Thomas Aquinas, but many other philosophers and theologians held it as well. (29) Natural law theory continued into the early Modern period, being found in the writings of such philosophers as Thomas Hobbes (30) and John Locke. (31) Among all the theories that go under the name of natural law, there is a common core of beliefs; namely, that the basic principles of morals and legislation are, in some sense or other, objective, accessible to reason, and based on human nature. (29)

In its classic form as presented by Aquinas, natural law ethics holds that what is in accord with human nature is to be considered right, and what goes against human nature is to be considered wrong. More exactly, we find that human nature has certain properties. These properties entail that a human being ought to do acts *a*, *b*, and *c* and ought not to do acts *x*, *y*, and *z*. (29) For example, we find that human beings have a natural inclination to self-preservation. What is in accord with self-preservation is right. It is right to exercise regularly in order to keep in shape physically since this promotes self-preservation. On the other hand, assisted suicide and euthanasia go against the natural inclination to self-preservation, and hence are judged ethically wrong actions.

Natural law has been used by the Catholic Church in evaluating assisted reproductive technologies. For example, the Catholic Church has used natural law reasoning to rule out the use of in vitro fertilization. What occurs naturally is that the act of sexual intercourse has two functions. It is an expression of love between two people (unitive purpose) but it is also the means by which children are conceived (procreative purpose). It is "unnatural" to separate the conception of a child from an interpersonal act of sexual intercourse, but by fertilizing an ovum in a dish in a laboratory, this is precisely what in vitro fertilization does. Hence, according to natural law ethics, in vitro fertilization is to be judged morally impermissible. (32)

A point presented in favor of natural law theory is that it provides a basis from which to address all people, without regard to their particular religious tradition. (33) This is so because it bases right and wrong on a human nature common to all people. On the other hand, the question is raised of exactly what "human nature" is. Historically, the nature of human beings has been conceived of in different ways. Some have emphasized reason as what is most characteristic of human beings; others have emphasized free will. Darwinians emphasize the continuity of human with non-human species. In the twentieth century, the existentialist philosopher Jean-Paul Sartre went so far as to deny that there is a "given" human nature, maintaining that human beings themselves are in the process of creating what a human is. (34)

Another criticism leveled against natural law theory pertains especially to the area of sexual ethics; namely, that it has a physicalist or biologistic bias, and does not give sufficient attention to the personal dimension of human beings. (33). This criticism might be leveled against the aforementioned judgment on in vitro fertilization which rules out the use of IVF because it separates the conception of a child from the act of sexual intercourse. This position has been criticized on the grounds that it places too much emphasis on the conjugal act as such (the physical, the biological) and not enough emphasis on the interpersonal love relationship between two people which provides the overall context for the use of IVF to have a child. (35)

Finally, it should be noted that certain principles of relevance to health care ethics have also come out of the natural law tradition, such as the principle of double effect. Basically, this principle justifies taking a course of action that has two types of effects: one effect is perfectly good and is what is wanted, while the other effect is bad and is not wanted but may accompany the first. (36) For example, among those opposed to abortion, the principle of double effect has been used to justify the removal of a cancerous uterus when a woman is pregnant. The desired effect is the removal of a diseased organ, which is a perfectly legitimate aim. In the case of pregnancy, however, removing the cancerous uterus will also mean the death of the fetus. The woman who is pregnant may not want to lose the child she is carrying, but this will be an unavoidable effect of removing the diseased organ. (36)

In its fully developed form, the principle of double effect includes the following stipulations: the act itself must be morally good or neutral, only the good consequences of the act must be intended, the good effect must not be produced by means of the evil effect, and there must be some weighty reason for permitting the evil. (37) For example, the act of removing a diseased organ, such as a cancerous uterus, is at least morally neutral and very possibly can be considered a morally good action. If a woman feels a loss because of the death of her child, it is clear that it is only the good consequence of removing a diseased organ which is intended by her, not the evil effect of the death of the child. If the cancerous uterus is removed with the fetus in it (rather than the fetus being killed before the removal of the uterus), then the evil effect of the death of the child is not the means of achieving the good effect. Finally, saving the life of the woman by removing a cancerous organ is certainly a weighty reason for permitting the evil of the death of her fetus.

Traditionally, the principle of double effect has been used to justify the administration of pain medication that may have a side effect of hastening death. (37) While almost everyone would agree that this course of action is morally permissible, not everyone would accept the principle of double effect as an appropriate justification for this action. This principle holds that death cannot be used as the means of relieving suffering but that it can be accepted as merely a foreseeable consequence of relieving suffering. Some have taken issue with this distinction, maintaining that "people are equally responsible for all of the foreseeable effects of their actions." (37) They see the real ethical issue as "whether or not the decision makers have considered the full range of foreseeable effects, have knowingly accepted whatever risk of death is entailed, and have found the risk to be justified in light of the paucity and undesirability of other options." (37)

Ethical Relativism vs. Ethical Objectivism

It is an undeniable fact that different groups of people—different societies, cultures, and subcultures—differ in their ethical judgments. For example, Hindus attribute a sacred status to cows, and consider it wrong to kill and eat them. (38) On the other hand, raising cattle for food is a major industry in the United States. Some Islamic traditions require a woman to wear a burka, an outer garment that cloaks the entire body, in public. This is done for the sake of promoting modesty in dress and behavior in public. (39) Mormon fundamentalist sects allow the practice of "plural marriage," a form of polygamy in which a man may have many wives. Mainline Mormons, on the other hand, practice monogamy. (40) Or again, just consider the vigorous debates over abortion and homosexuality in the United States!

The fact of disagreement in ethical judgments has promoted the position known as *ethical relativism.* Ethical relativism denies that there is a single, objectively true moral standard that is valid for everyone everywhere. The relativist maintains that what is right and wrong varies among different cultures and societies. (41) Thus, according to the relativist, euthanasia and assisted suicide may be morally right in one culture but wrong in another. In making this claim, the relativist is not speaking merely of what people may think is right or wrong, because people can make mistakes in their moral judgments. Rather, the relativist is asserting that what in fact is right or wrong varies among different cultures and societies.

Ethical relativism is *not* itself an ethical theory or principle. Rather, it makes a claim *about* ethical theories and principles. It claims that no ethical theory or principle holds good for everyone everywhere. According to the relativist, utilitarianism may be an appropriate ethical theory for one society, but not for another. The principle of patient autonomy may be right for North Americans but not for Asians.

The West has sometimes suffered from *ethnocentrism,* the belief that its culture is inherently superior to other cultures. (41) Such a view has been condemned "as a variety of prejudice tantamount to racism and sexism." (41) A reaction to ethnocentrism is a movement "not to judge others but to be tolerant of diversity." (41) Ethical relativism seems to fit with such an "attitude of tolerance toward other cultures." (41)

Some philosophers, however, have argued that ethical relativism has implications that go against common sense and common practice. These unacceptable implications are reasons for judging ethical relativism to be incorrect.

For one thing, ethical relativism prevents us from ever criticizing the practices of another society as evil:

Suppose a society waged war on its neighbors for the purpose of taking slaves. Or suppose a society was violently anti-Semitic, and its leaders set out to destroy the Jews. Cultural Relativism would preclude us from saying that either of these practices was wrong. We would not even be able to say that a society tolerant of Jews is *better* than the anti-Semitic society, for that would imply some sort of transcultural standard of comparison. The failure to condemn *these* practices does not seem "enlightened"; on the contrary, slavery and anti-Semitism seem wrong *wherever* they occur. Nevertheless, if we took Cultural Relativism seriously, we would have to admit that these social practices also are immune from criticism. (42)

These societal practices would be immune from criticism precisely because what is right and wrong is determined by the particular society.

Moreover, ethical relativism destroys our notion of social reform. For relativism "seems to entail that reformers are always (morally) wrong, because they go against the cultural tide." (41) However, "we normally feel just the opposite: that the reformer is the courageous innovator who is right, who has the truth, against the mindless majority." (41)

Further, ethical relativism destroys the notion of moral progress. This point can be illustrated by the changing status of women in society:

> Usually, we think that at least some changes in our society have been for the better. . . . Throughout most of Western history the place of women in society was very narrowly circumscribed. They could not own property; they could not vote or hold political office; with a few exceptions, they were not permitted to have paying jobs; and generally they were under the almost absolute control of their husbands. Recently much of this has changed, and most people think of it as progress.
>
> If Cultural Relativism is correct, can we legitimately think of this as progress? Progress means replacing a way of doing things with a *better* way. But by what standard do we judge the new ways as better? If the old ways were in accordance with the social standards of their time, then Cultural Relativism would say it is a mistake to judge them by the standards of a different time. Eighteenth-century society was, in effect, a different society from the one we have now. To say that we have made progress implies a judgment that present-day society is better, and that is just the sort of transcultural judgment that, according to Cultural Relativism, is impermissible. (42)

However, it does make sense to think that our society has made some moral progress. Because ethical relativism "says that these judgments make no sense," so the argument goes, "it cannot be right." (42)

According to ethical relativism, right and wrong are determined by a culture or society. This contention entails yet another problem because "one person may belong to several societies (subcultures) with different value emphases and arrangements of principles." (41) For example, "if Mary is a U.S. citizen and a member of the Roman Catholic Church, she is wrong (as a Catholic) if she chooses to have an abortion and not wrong (as a U.S. citizen) if she acts against the teaching of the Church on abortion." (41) According to relativism, just what is the ethically right thing for Mary to do?

In sum, there are serious problems with ethical relativism. The alternative view is ethical objectivism, the position that there are some ethical principles—at least, some basic or core ethical principles—that are valid for everyone everywhere. (43) But then how does one account for the diversity of ethical judgments actually found in our world? Here is one explanation:

> Consider a culture in which people believe it is wrong to eat cows. This may even be a poor culture, in which there is not enough food; still, the cows are not to be touched. Such a society would *appear* to have values very different from our own. But does it? We have not yet asked why these people will not eat cows. Suppose it is because they believe that after death the souls of humans inhabit the bodies of animals, especially cows, so that a cow may be someone's grandmother. Now do we want to say that their values are different from ours? No, the difference lies elsewhere. The difference is in our belief systems, not in our values. We agree that we shouldn't eat Grandma; we simply disagree about whether the cow *is* (or could be) Grandma. (42)

In other words, opponents of ethical relativism claim that different cultures and societies may share the same basic moral principles and values but put these principles and values into practice in different ways because of different factual beliefs. Or again, the same principles and values may be put into practice in different ways because of different circumstances. For example, it has been suggested that Eskimos kill perfectly normal infants *not* because they have less affection for their children or less respect for human life than we do, but for reasons having to do with their lifestyle and survival. Eskimo mothers will nurse their children for four years, which places limits on the number of infants that one mother can sustain. In addition, Eskimos are nomadic since they are unable to farm, and a mother can carry only one baby as she travels. (42)

While flaws are apparent in ethical relativism, can anything be said positively in favor of ethical objectivism? It has been argued that "there are some moral rules that all societies will have in common, because those rules are necessary for society to exist." (42) A prohibition against lying is given as one example:

> Imagine what it would be like for a society to place no value at all on truth telling. When one person spoke to another, there would be no

presumption at all that he was telling the truth—for he could just as easily be speaking falsely. Within that society, there would be no reason to pay attention to what anyone says. (I ask you what time it is, and you say "four o'clock." But there is no presumption that you are speaking truly; you could just as easily have said the first thing that came into your head. So I have no reason to pay attention to your answer—in fact, there was no point in my asking you in the first place!) Communication would then be extremely difficult, if not impossible. And because complex societies cannot exist without regular communication among their members, society would become impossible. It follows that in any complex society there *must* be a presumption in favor of truthfulness. There may of course be exceptions to this rule: there may be situations in which it is thought to be permissible to lie. Nevertheless, these will be exceptions to a rule that *is* in force in the society. (42)

The prohibition against murder is given as another example of a rule needed for a society to survive. (42) One philosopher has developed the following list of core moral principles binding on all human beings:

1. It is morally wrong to torture people for the fun of it.
2. Do not kill innocent people.
3. Do not cause pain or suffering except when a higher duty prescribes it.
4. Do not commit rape.
5. Keep your promises and contracts.
6. Do not deprive another person of his or her freedom.
7. Do justice, treating equals equally and unequals unequally.
8. Tell the truth.
9. Help other people.
10. Obey just laws. (41)

Among these allegedly common moral principles, [2], [3], [5], [7], [8] and [9] have definite implications for the field of health care.

References

1. Diane E. Hoffmann, Philip Boyle & Steven A. Levenson, *Handbook for Nursing Home Ethics Committees* (Washington, DC: American Association of Homes and Services for the Aging, 1995).

2. Patrick Norris, OP, "The McCaughey Septuplets: All's Well that Ends Well?" *Health Care Ethics USA* (Spring 1998): 6-7.
3. Michael D. Lemonick, "It's a Miracle," *Time* (December 1, 1997): 34-39.
4. Tom L. Beauchamp and James F. Childress, *Principles of Biomedical Ethics*, 5th ed. (New York: Oxford, 2001).
5. Judith Wilson Ross, John W, Glaser, Dorothy Rasinki-Gregory, Joan McIver Gibson, and Corrine Bayley, *Health Care Ethics Committees The Next Generation* (Chicago: American Hospital Publishing, 1993).
6. "Principles of Distributive Justice" in Ronald Munson (ed.), *Intervention and Reflection Basic Issues in Medical Ethics*, 8th ed. (Belmont, CA: Thomson Wadsworth, 2008).
7. Maureen Weaver, Jeanette C. Schreiber, Michelle Wilcox DeBarge, Catherine P. Baatz, Wiggin & Dana, LLP, *The HIPAA Handbook Implementing the Federal Privacy Rule in the Long-Term Care Setting* (Washington, DC: American Association of Homes and Services for the Aging, 2001).
8. Office of Civil Rights, *Standards for Privacy of Individually Identifiable Health Information,* http://www.hhs.gov/ocr/hipaa/finalmaster.html. Accessed 2002.
9. Robert N. Bellah, Richard Madsen, William M. Sullivan, Ann Swidler, and Steven M. Tipton, *Habits of the Heart* (New York: Harper & Row, 1985).
10. Celia Wolf-Devine, "Abortion and the 'Feminine Voice,'" *Public Affairs Quarterly* 3/3 (July 1989): 81-97.
11. "Normative Theories of Ethics" in William H. Shaw (ed.), *Social and Personal Ethics*, 2nd ed. (Belmont, CA: Wadsworth, 1996).
12. Jeremy Bentham, *An Introduction to the Principles of Morals and Legislation* in *The Utilitarians* (Garden City, NY: Anchor/Doubleday, 1973).
13. John Stuart Mill, *Utilitarianism* (Indianapolis: Bobbs-Merrill, 1957).
14. Wikipedia, s.v. "Utilitarianism," http://en.wikipedia.org/wiki/Utilitarianism. Accessed April 2009.
15. "Reproductive Control" in Ronald Munson (ed.), *Intervention and Reflection: Basic Issues in Medical Ethics*, 8th ed. (Belmont, CA: Thomson Wadsworth, 2008).
16. Heidi Malm, "Paid Surrogacy: Arguments and Responses," *Public Affairs Quarterly* 3/2 (April 1989): 57-66.
17. Elizabeth S. Anderson, "Is Women's Labor a Commodity?" *Philosophy and Public Affairs* 19/1 (Winter 1990): 71-87, 90-92.
18. Jonathan Harrison, "Utilitarianism, Universalization, and Our Duty to Be Just," *Proceedings of the Aristotelian Society* 53 (1952-3): 105-34.
19. "Utilitarianism" in Ronald Munson (ed.), *Intervention and Reflectio Issues in Medical Ethics*, 8th ed. (Belmont, CA: Thomson Wadsw

20. "Ethical Theories: Autonomy, Truth Telling, Confidentiality" in Ronald Munson (ed.), *Intervention and Reflection: Basic Issues in Medical Ethics,* 8th ed. (Belmont, CA: Thomson Wadsworth, 2008).
21. Martin Curd, *Argument and Analysis An Introduction to Philosophy* (St. Paul: West, 1992).
22. W.D. Ross, *The Right and the Good* (Oxford: Oxford University Press, 1930).
23. Kai Nielsen, "A Defense of Utilitarianism," *Ethics* 82 (1972): 113-24.
24. Immanuel Kant, *The Foundations of the Metaphysics of Morals,* trans. T.K. Abbott in William H. Shaw (ed.), *Social and Personal Ethics,* 2nd ed. (Belmont, CA: Wadsworth, 1996).
25. Ruth Macklin, "Is There Anything Wrong with Surrogate Motherhood? An Ethical Analysis," *Law, Medicine & Health Care* 16 (1988): 57-64.
26. *Human Experiments: The Price of Knowledge?* KCTS/Seattle, 1980, video.
27. William K. Frankena, *Ethics,* 2nd ed. (Englewood Cliffs, NJ: Prentice-Hall, 1973).
28. "Ross's Ethics" in Ronald Munson (ed.), *Intervention and Reflection: Basic Issues in Medical Ethics,* 8th ed. (Belmont, CA: Thomson Wadsworth, 2008).
29. D.J. O'Connor, *Aquinas and Natural Law* (London: Macmillan, 1967).
30. Thomas Hobbes, *Leviathan* (New York: E.P. Dutton, 1950).
31. John Locke, *Essays on the Law of Nature,* trans. W. von Leyden (Oxford: Clarendon, 1965).
32. Vatican Congregation for the Doctrine of the Faith, *Instruction on Respect for Human Life in its Origin and On the Dignity of Procreation* (Washington, DC: United States Catholic Conference, 1987).
33. James F. Gustafson, *Protestant and Roman Catholic Ethics: Prospects for Rapprochement* (Chicago: University of Chicago Press, 1978).
34. *What is Human Nature?* Insight Media, video.
35. Ethics Committee of the American Fertility Society, "Ethical Consideration of the New Reproductive Technologies" in Richard T. Hull (ed.), *Ethical Issues in the New Reproductive Technologies* (Belmont, CA: Wadsworth, 1990).
36. Orville N. Griese, *Catholic Identity in Health Care: Principles and Practice* (Braintree, MA: Pope John Center, 1987).
37. President's Commission for the Study of Ethical Problems in Medicine and Biomedical and Behavioral Research, *Deciding to Forego Life-Sustaining Treatment* (1983; reprint New York: Concern for Dying).
38. Religionfacts, *The Cow in Hinduism.* http://www.religionfacts.com/hinduism/things/cow.htm. Accessed April 2009.
39. Wikipedia, s.v. Burqa. http://en.wikipedia.org/wiki/Burqa. Accessed April 2009.

40. Wikipedia, s.v. Mormon fundamentalism. http://en.wikipedia.org/wiki/Morman_Fundamentalism. Accessed April 2009.
41. Louis Pojman, "Ethical Relativism versus Ethical Objectivism" in Louis P. Pojman, *Introduction to Philosophy: Classical and Contemporary Readings* (Belmont, CA: Wadsworth, 1991).
42. James Rachels, "The Challenge of Cultural Relativism" in Joel Feinberg, *Reason and Responsibility: Readings in Some Basic Problems of Philosophy,* 9th ed. (Belmont, CA: Wadsworth, 1996).
43. Louis Pojman, "A Critique of Ethical Relativism" in Louis Pojman (ed.), *Ethical Theory Classical and Contemporary Readings,* 3rd ed. (Belmont, CA: Wadsworth, 1998).

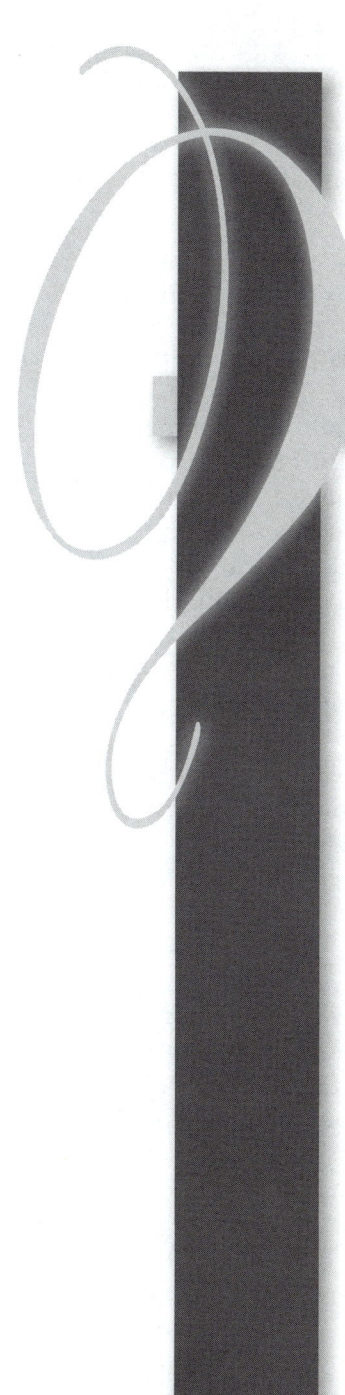

Chapter 2

Ethics Committees: A Resource for Resolving Ethical Dilemmas

Many of the most puzzling questions faced today by health care providers and by patients and their families are not exclusively medical in character, but involve individual and institutional values. Ethics committees raise consciousness about the moral dimensions of health care decision making and provide a forum for working through difficult ethical problems.

While ethics committees began in the acute care, hospital setting, they have expanded to long-term care facilities and other types of health care services. Initially ethics committees focused on issues in *clinical practice*. They discussed, for example, when it is permissible to withhold or withdraw life-sustaining treatments. Some committees have expanded the scope of their activity to include *organizational ethics,* considering administrative, financial, and human resource questions. (1) In fact, some facilities have established separate clinical and organizational ethics committees. In this book we will focus on the work of ethics committees in a clinical context.

Functions of an Ethics Committee

An ethics committee typically has three functions: education, the development and review of institutional policies and guidelines, and case consultation.

One of the primary functions of an ethics committee is providing education on issues in health care ethics. This includes education of the committee members themselves, who come from a variety of professional backgrounds. It also includes continuing education and in-service programs for health care providers within the facility. In addition, ethics committees engage in community education, developing programming for the general public.

Second, ethics committees are involved in developing and reviewing policies and guidelines for the facility that have an ethical dimension. For example, an ethics committee may assist in developing a policy on futile medical treatment to be sent to the facility's medical staff and/or board for approval. Or the committee may be asked to review and revise a policy that is already in place on the use of restraints.

Third, an ethics committee is typically available for consultation with patients, family members, and health care providers about difficult ethical dilemmas they face. This committee activity will later be described at length.

The Make-Up of an Ethics Committee

Ethics committees usually have between twelve and fifteen members. The membership is multidisciplinary, representing various types of work in health care and various professions. The committee is not necessarily composed entirely of employees of the facility; it may include some individuals from within the community the facility serves.

An ethics committee, whether at a hospital or a long-term care facility, typically includes representation from the following groups:

- board of trustees;
- administration;
- medical staff (physicians);
- nursing staff;
- clergy/pastoral care staff;
- social workers;

- attorneys;
- ethicists (usually, philosophy or theology professors);
- patient advocates (for example, parent of a disabled child, member of handicapped persons' association, resident of a long-term care facility).

However, this does not preclude membership by other types of health care professionals. Consistent with the concept of an integrated community health care system, an ethics committee may also include representatives from such areas as pharmacy, allied health, hospice services, home health care, adult day care, and assisted living services.

Many ethics committees serve just one particular facility. However, a number of facilities in a particular geographical area will sometimes join together to establish a regional ethics committee serving all the participating facilities. Some ethics committees meet monthly, others meet bi-monthly, and yet others meet only quarterly.

Ethics Consultation

Patients and family members can discuss the ethical dimensions of treatment decisions with their health care providers or with pastoral care staff. Health care providers can talk with co-workers. However, a time may come when patients, family, or health care providers feel that they have reached the limits of their own abilities to address an ethical issue. In such cases an ethics consult may be a helpful resource.

An *ethics consult* is a meeting with members of the ethics committee to work through difficult issues in patient care from the point of view of moral rightness and wrongness. Sometimes the whole ethics committee will be involved, sometimes a subcommittee of it.

An ethics consult may

- provide information about ethical principles relevant to the case under discussion;
- help clarify what options are open;
- provide information about similar cases;
- provide information about relevant policies of the facility;
- result in recommendations that are advisory in nature.

Ethics consultation services are not intended to replace the normal lines of communication among health care providers, patients, and families. But an ethics consult may be helpful when

- a patient, family member, or health care provider wants help in "talking through" ethical issues involved in patient care;
- there is a serious ethical disagreement between health care providers, among family members, between health care providers and the patient, or between health care providers and family members;
- ethically, the case is unusual, unprecedented, or very complex;
- a patient, family member, or health care provider would like to have the benefit of other perspectives in working through an ethical problem.

Any recommendations made by the consultants are purely advisory in nature. Patients, family members, and health care providers remain responsible for making their own decisions.

A notation that an ethics consult has taken place may be put into the patient's medical record. Ethics consults are treated as confidential. They may subsequently be discussed by the members of the ethics committee, but with appropriate safeguards for maintaining confidentiality. (2)

In this book students will be invited to role play membership on an ethics committee.

References

1. Judith Wilson Ross, et al., *Health Care Ethics Committees The Next Generation* (Chicago: American Hospital Publishing, 1993).
2. The information on ethics consultation is adapted from brochures prepared by the Clinical Ethics Committee of Mercy Medical Center, Dubuque, Iowa and the Medical Ethics Committee of the University of Nebraska Medical Center.

Part One

Ethical Issues at the Beginning of Life

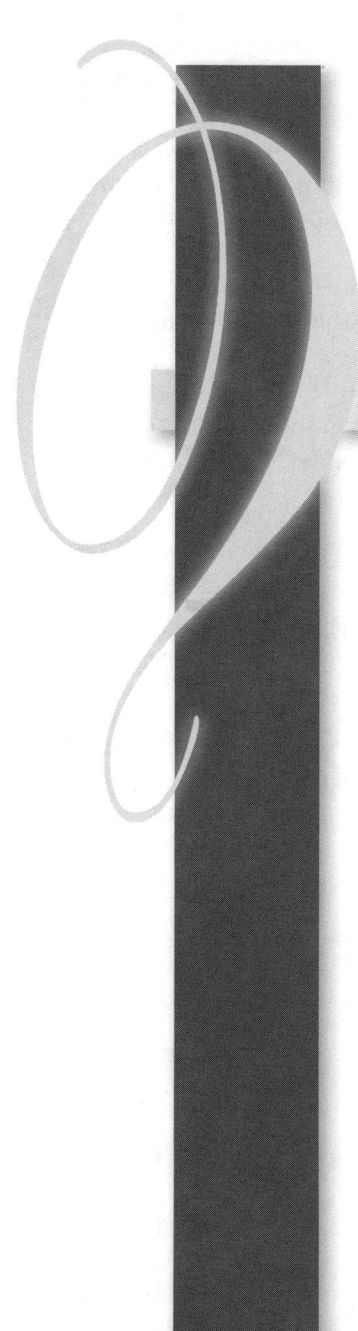

Chapter 3

The Abortion Debate

Ever since the *Roe v. Wade* decision of the United States Supreme Court in 1973 legalizing the practice of abortion, abortion has been one of the most divisive issues in American society. People regularly categorize themselves as being either "pro-choice" or "pro-life."

Abortion may be defined as "the termination of a pregnancy with resulting death of the human fetus." (1) So defined, the term abortion is a generic term covering a number of different events and procedures. A distinction can be made between *spontaneous abortion*, which is another name for a miscarriage, and *induced* or *procured abortion*, which is caused by human action. Within the category of induced or procured abortions, a distinction can be made between *indirect* and *direct abortions*. An indirect abortion occurs when the direct, immediate purpose of the procedure is to treat the mother for a threatening pathology, but the death of the fetus is also an inevitable result (which would have been avoided if possible). An example of an indirect abortion is surgery to remove a cancerous uterus when a woman is pregnant. On the other hand, a direct abortion occurs when the direct, immediate purpose of the procedure is to destroy the human fetus or to expel it when it is not viable. (1) Ethically, what is controversial is the practice of direct abortion, and it is this type of abortion that will be the focus of the present chapter. When the term "abortion" is used in this chapter, it will be understood as referring to "direct abortion."

Three different positions have been taken on the morality of abortion. First, there is the position of *abortion on demand,* which is the view that abortion is permissible at any time during a pregnancy for any reason whatever. A second position would allow *abortion in a limited number of cases;* for example, in cases of rape or incest, or when the fetus is suffering from a severe abnormality, or when the pregnancy threatens the well-being (physical or psychological) of the mother. The third position is that *abortion is never permissible.*

In this chapter you will learn about:

- common arguments for and against the ethical permissibility of abortion;
- the controversy about when human life begins;
- selective abortion in the case of fetal abnormality;
- preimplantation genetic diagnosis;
- abortion in the case of rape.

Case Study

Connie and Roger Young are in their mid-thirties and have been married for eleven years. They have two children, Julie, 8, and Melissa, 6. Now that the children are older and in school, Connie has resumed teaching full-time. Roger respects Connie's desire to pursue her own career. Besides, they can use the second income.

Barbara Cullen works as a speech and hearing therapist in the school system in which Connie teaches. Barbara and Connie have been good friends for some time. Lately, Barbara can tell that Connie has been agitated and upset.

One day when they are having lunch together, Barbara asks Connie what is wrong. Connie confesses that she has recently learned that she is pregnant—unexpectedly and unintentionally. She and Roger had decided they would have two children—no more. She had been using a diaphragm for birth control, but obviously it didn't provide one hundred percent protection. Roger, she says, has been trying to take a positive attitude towards having another child. Indeed, he has joked that maybe this time they will have the son he has always wanted!

Connie, on the other hand, is very concerned about what the birth of another child will do to her developing career. Further, having another child will put a strain on the family's financial resources, and she doubts that this is really fair to the welfare of the children they already have. Connie has told Roger that she feels she has to have an abortion. Roger, she tells Barbara, didn't like that at all.

Connie does not like to do something against the wishes of her husband. So far, their marriage has been a good one. At the same time, she feels strongly that she should have the final say about the abortion. After all, it is her body and her life that is at stake.

Barbara has befriended some of the girls at school who have become pregnant, and tried to encourage them to think about and work through some of the ethical issues surrounding abortion before they rush into having one. She wonders if she should take the same approach with her co-worker Connie.

■ ■ ■

Common Arguments For and Against the Permissibility of Abortion

Personalizing common arguments in the abortion debate to the case of Connie Young, the following considerations might be brought forward in support of Connie's choice to have an abortion:

- Connie will have to bear the risk and burden of pregnancy, delivery, and child care. It will be extremely difficult for her to undergo this unless it is her choice to do so. (1)
- Connie has the right to a normal sex life, on which her marriage and the care of her other children also depend. Since artificial contraception does not give her complete control over pregnancy, she has the right to use abortion as a last resort. (1)
- Connie has the right to control what happens to her body because it is her property. If a pregnancy occurs unintentionally and accidentally, the fetus

can be compared to a trespasser on the woman's property who has no right to the use of her body. (2)
- For Connie to bear an unwanted child will be a disaster for the child as well as for Connie. No matter how hard she may try, Connie may not be able to provide the child with the kind of atmosphere the child needs psychologically, and may even engage in child neglect or abuse. (1)

On the other hand, the following arguments might be offered against Connie having an abortion:

- While continuing with the pregnancy may cause certain hardships for Connie, these hardships are not as severe as what the fetus suffers through abortion; namely, the complete loss of life. The fetus's right to life takes precedence over the avoidance of hardships for Connie. (1)
- Everyone should realize that no method of birth control, other than abstinence, is one hundred percent effective. By voluntarily engaging in sexual relations, Connie has given the fetus the right to use her body.
- Even if a woman's body is her property, this does not give her any right to kill a fetus within her body. In general, ownership of property does not give one the right to kill innocent people who are on, or even trespassing on, one's property. In fact, a property owner can be held responsible if people injure themselves while on his property. (3)
- By having an abortion, Connie is guilty of taking an innocent human life.
- Having an abortion is not likely to relieve Connie of stress and give her peace of mind. Women who have abortions may later experience psychological repercussions for which they may have to seek counseling.
- As partly responsible for its existence, Roger also has rights concerning what is done with the fetus. In having an abortion contrary to Roger's wishes, Connie is ignoring and violating Roger's rights as a father.

The claim that abortion is wrong because it is an act of killing a human being is a major argument in the abortion debate. It deserves special attention.

The Controversy about the Beginning of Human Life

More formally stated, the argument at issue is this: Killing an innocent human being is ethically wrong; because abortion takes the life of an innocent human being, abortion must be considered ethically wrong.

The first premise of this argument, "Killing an innocent human being is ethically wrong," contains a qualification about "innocence." This qualification is meant to establish a distinction from the case of capital punishment in which an evildoer is killed. The second premise of the argument, "Abortion takes the life of an innocent human being," assumes that the fetus is a human being. This, in turn, raises the question of exactly when human life begins.

In *Roe v. Wade,* the 1973 U.S. Supreme Court decision legalizing abortion, the Court saw viability as the critical time in the pregnancy, after which there might be governmental regulation and even prohibition of abortion. (4) Viability is the time at which a fetus can be removed from the mother's womb and live apart from her, perhaps with some technological assistance. (4) At viability, the fetus has existence independent of the mother, and this is the reason it is taken as the beginning of an individual human life.

However, viability is not an absolutely fixed point, and this poses a problem for selecting it as the beginning of a human life. For one thing, the time of viability depends on the state of our technology. At the time of the *Roe v. Wade* decision in 1973, viability was placed at twenty-eight weeks. (5) However, by the 1980s, advances in neonatal care made twenty-four weeks the generally accepted dividing line. (5) Indeed, "the perfection of artificial incubation may make the fetus viable at any time." (6) Moreover, mere length of life of the fetus is not an exact measure of viability.

> Perinatologists (specialists in newborns) say that too many factors are involved in determining viability to make reliable generalizations about which fetuses will live and which will die at any given stage of development. In addition to characteristics such as a fetus's weight and the developmental stage of the organs, factors like the health of the mother, her socioeconomic status, and her access to health care also play a role. So do the race and the gender of the fetus. In development, a white fetus generally lags a week behind an African American one of the same age, and a male fetus lags the same amount behind a female. (7)

In sum, "if viability is the norm, the standard would vary with race and with many individual circumstances." (6) And if there is so much variability in viability, then viability does not seem to provide a secure basis for determining the time when human life begins.

Others push the beginning of human life back to the time of conception/fertilization. Within this camp, some see a human being coming into existence as soon as the sperm has entered and united with the ovum; others see syngamy as the definitive point, when the nuclei of the ovum and the sperm have fused to form a new, single nucleus with a complete set of chromosomes. (1, 8) The following biological facts about the embryo are cited to support classifying it as a human being from the time of conception/fertilization:

> First, the embryo is from the start distinct from any cell of the mother or of the father. This is clear because it is growing in its own distinct direction. Its growth is internally directed to its own survival and maturation. Second, the embryo is human: it has the genetic makeup characteristic of human beings. Third, and most important, the embryo is a complete or whole organism, though immature. The human embryo, from conception onwards, is fully programmed and has the active disposition to use that information to develop himself or herself to the mature stage of a human being, and, unless prevented by disease or violence, will actually do so.... None of the changes that occur to the embryo after fertilization, for as long as he or she survives, generates a new direction of growth.... Rather, all of the changes... either facilitate or retard the internally directed growth of this determinate and enduring individual. (8)

Thus it is asserted that "a human embryo is not something different in kind from a human being, like a rock, or a potato, or a rhinoceros." (8) Rather, "a human embryo is a whole living member of the species Homo sapiens in the earliest stage of his or her natural development." (8)

One challenge to regarding conception/fertilization as the beginning of human life is found in our criteria for determining death. The irreversible cessation of brain activity is one of the accepted criteria of death. (9) Therefore, by symmetry, should not the beginning of brain activity be taken as the beginning of human life? Brain activity usually becomes detectable in the fetus during the eighth week, and the brain structure is complete at twelve weeks. (8, 10)

Those espousing the position that human life begins at the time of conception/fertilization offer the following reply to this challenge:

> ... brain death is accepted because the irreversible collapse of the brain destroys the capacity for self-directed integral organic functioning of human beings who have matured to the stage at which the brain performs the key role in integrating the organism....
>
> By contrast, although an embryo has not yet developed a brain, its capacity to do so is inherent and developing.... Moreover, the embryo is clearly exercising self-directed integral organic functioning, and so is a unitary organism.... A factor or factors other than the brain makes possible its self-integration and organic functioning. (8)

In other words, it is suggested that what is needed for human life to exist is "self-directed integral organic functioning." This function is performed by the brain but, in the case of the embryo and early stage fetus, it is achieved by other physiological factors.

However, several biological facts about human reproduction are also brought forward against regarding conception/fertilization as the beginning point of a particular human life: twinning, embryo fusion, and natural wastage.

During the first two weeks after conception/fertilization, the embryo can split to form identical (monozygotic) twins, or even triplets or higher order multiples. (11) This possibility provides evidence that "the early embryo is not yet one human being, but a community of possibly different individuals held together by a gelatinous membrane." (11) Moreover, it sometimes happens that "separate and genetically distinct embryos (which might have gone on to become fraternal twins) fuse during early development to form a single human being." (11) Hence, until the time for twinning and embryo recombination has passed, we do not know how many human beings are actually present. And until we know how many individuals are present, how can we speak of the beginning of their human life? Thus the phenomena of twinning and embryo fusion have led some to conclude that biological individuality is not established until the time of gastrulation, which begins at two weeks of gestational age. (11)

In the case of twinning, the following reply has been made by those supporting conception/fertilization as the beginning of a human life:

> Consider the parallel case of division of a flatworm. Parts of a flatworm have the potential to become a whole flatworm when isolated from the present whole of which they are a part. Yet no one would suggest that prior to the division of a flatworm to produce two whole flatworms, the original flatworm was not a unitary individual.
>
> Likewise, at the early stages of human embryonic development, before specialization by the cells has progressed very far, the cells or groups of cells can become whole organisms if they are divided and have an appropriate environment after the division. But that fact does not in the least indicate that prior to such an extrinsic division the embryo is other than a unitary, self-integrating, actively developing human organism. (8)

Further, with respect to embryo recombination, it is admitted that the frequency of occurrence of this phenomenon within the human population has not been precisely determined. (11)

Natural wastage is another biological fact that has been seen to cast doubt on conception/fertilization as the beginning of human life:

> Reproductive embryologists report that human embryos have a very high natural rate of mortality during the first few weeks of development. Estimates vary greatly, but some studies suggest that in normal healthy women, between two-thirds and three-quarters of all fertilized eggs do not go on to implant in the womb. Some of this embryonic loss results from complex biological processes that screen embryos for genetic or chromosomal abnormalities. Embryos that fail to pass this test are sloughed off as a late menstrual period, often without any awareness on the woman's part that she was pregnant. . . . In view of this high rate of embryonic loss, do we truly want to bestow much moral significance on an entity with which nature is so wasteful? (11)

In reply, it has been pointed out that, since a number of these unsuccessful pregnancies are actually due to chromosomal defects, "it seems plausible to infer that in some cases, these defects are so significant that a human embryo probably failed to form." (8) In other words, "in some, and perhaps many cases, what is lost is not an embryo but a nonembryonic entity resulting from defects in the fertilization process." (8)

As noted in the *Roe v. Wade* decision, "those trained in the respective disciplines of medicine, philosophy, and theology" have not yet been able to "arrive at any consensus" about exactly when human life begins. (4) However, it might be argued that, even if the fetus is not human until some point in development later than conception/fertilization, it is still the case that there is the *potential* for human life from the time of conception/fertilization. This potential for human life, it might be claimed, makes the developing embryo and fetus different from a mere clump of cells, and entitles its life to be protected.

Human Being vs. Human Person

Another twist in the abortion debate is to acknowledge that an embryo is a human being, but to make a distinction between a "human being" and a "human person" with the accompanying claim that it is only human "persons" who have rights, including a right to life. (8) Characteristics that have been suggested as constituting "persons" include self-consciousness (of oneself as existing over time), a capacity to act on reasons, a capacity to communicate with others using a language, a capacity to act freely, and rationality. (12) The claim is that, according to this standard, embryos and fetuses do not display the requisite cognitive characteristics to qualify as human "persons" and hence cannot be accorded a "right to life."

Several arguments have been offered against the plausibility of this position. First, proponents of this view "do not wish…to exclude from the status of 'persons' human beings who are asleep or who are in reversible comas" (8), so that the cognitive abilities in question must be construed as a "capacity or potentiality of some sort." (8) In other words, "sleeping or reversibly comatose human beings *are* persons because they have the potentiality or capacity for higher mental functions." (8) However, "human embryos and fetuses also possess, albeit in radical form, a capacity or potentiality for such mental functions." (8) Thus embryos and fetuses cannot be disqualified from the status of being human "persons."

Moreover, a developing human being does not display the cognitive characteristics in question until some time after birth. For example, "a six-week-old baby lacks the immediately or even nearly immediately exercisable capacity to perform characteristically human mental functions." (8) Hence, "if full moral respect were due only to those who possess a nearly immediately exercisable capacity for characteristically human mental functions, it would follow that six-week-old infants do not deserve full moral respect." (8) And thus, "if abortion were morally acceptable on the grounds that the human embryo or fetus lacks such a capacity for characteristically human mental functions, then one would be logically committed to the view that, subject to parental approval, human infants could be disposed of as well." (8) To reach such a conclusion is absurd.

Case Study

Anita and Sheila are sisters who have always been especially close. In fact, they married brothers, Robert and Allen. Anita got married first, followed by Sheila two years later. Both love children and have always wanted to have three or four each.

However, when Sheila becomes pregnant, she decides to have the health of her fetus checked through prenatal diagnosis. This is because her sister Anita has already given birth to a son with cystic fibrosis, an inheritable genetic disorder. An ultrasound reveals that Sheila is carrying twins. Amniocentesis gives her the bad news that both of her babies have cystic fibrosis.

Cystic fibrosis (CF) causes the body to produce thick, sticky mucus that clogs the lungs and leads to life-threatening infections. Because of this, therapy must be done with children with CF several times a day. Occasionally, they require hospitalization. There is currently no cure for cystic fibrosis. Some people with CF live into their thirties, but some die at a much younger age.

More than once Anita has telephoned Sheila crying because of the strains of caregiving. Because of her son's needs, Anita has had to give up her teaching job and feels confined to her home. Because of her sister's experience, Sheila is aware of the time demands of caring for a CF child, and the emotional strain of worrying about the child's future and of having to face the possibility of the child's death. Having the responsibility of one CF child is enough, but having two such children to care for is more than Sheila thinks she can deal with.

Cystic fibrosis is a recessive genetic disorder. Although Sheila and her husband themselves do not have CF, they must both be carriers of the gene for CF in order to have a child affected by cystic fibrosis. For each pregnancy there is a 25 percent chance of conceiving a child affected by CF, and a 75 percent chance of conceiving a child who will not be affected by this genetic disorder. Sheila talks with her husband about aborting the two fetuses with CF she is carrying, and starting another pregnancy in the hope of conceiving a healthy child. After all, she thinks, bad luck can't be with them forever!

■ ■ ■

Selective Abortion for Fetal Abnormalities

What is at issue in the case of Sheila's pregnancy is known as "selective abortion." It is not the case that an abortion is performed because no child is wanted. Rather, an abortion is performed only to prevent the birth of a particular kind of child; in this case, a child with a genetic disease.

As well as the arguments used to justify abortion in general, some special considerations are brought forward in support of the selective abortion of fetuses with abnormalities:

- *Aborting abnormal fetuses prevents suffering for the family.* Parents encounter rough spots in raising any child, but the strains are increased in caring for a child suffering from a serious disease. The strains are not only financial, but also emotional. (13)

- *Aborting an abnormal fetus prevents suffering for the child himself or herself.* Because of the suffering the disease would bring the child, giving life to the fetus would cause more harm to it than denying it life through abortion. Because of the poor quality of life the child would have if born, abortion can be seen as being in the best interests of the child himself or herself. (14)
- *Aborting abnormal fetuses benefits society as a whole.* Abortion brings about a substantial saving of societal resources that would otherwise be used for the special care and education of children suffering from serious diseases. These resources can be used for individuals who are able to make return contributions to society. (13)

It should be noted that these arguments are in accord with a *utilitarian* approach to ethics. (See chapter 1.) The utilitarian looks at consequences of actions in judging their rightness and wrongness, and maintains that the right action to perform is the one having the best consequences for everyone who will be affected by the action, including society as a whole.

Persons who are pro-life and opposed to abortion under any circumstances are likely to try to counter these arguments with the following points:

- With some diseases and disorders, the severity of the symptoms varies from individual to individual. For example, Down syndrome is a genetically based disorder which involves certain characteristic physical features (such as short stature, flat face, tongue protruding through thick lips) as well as mental impairment. However, the degree of mental impairment can range from severe to slight. (15) Even identical twins with cystic fibrosis can differ in how much they show the symptoms of the disease. (16) Prenatal diagnosis only indicates whether the child will be affected by a particular disease or disorder; it does not provide information about its severity. One could abort a child who would be only mildly affected by a disease or disorder.
- Even though a child suffers from a disease or disorder, he can still have a good quality of life. The disease or disorder is not the totality of the person. The child may have distinct abilities—artistic talents, wit, or intellect—that make life enjoyable for him as well as enabling him to contribute to society. (17) An example is Blaine Deatherage-Newsome who has spina bifida, is paralyzed from the armpits down, and is confined to a wheel chair; nevertheless, he was also an A student in high school and a national chess champion. (18) This is how Blaine describes his life:

> I was born with spina bifida and hydrocephalus. I hear that when parents have a test and find out that their unborn child has spina bifida, in

more than 95 percent of the cases they choose to have an abortion. I also went to an exhibit at the Oregon Museum of Science and Industry several years ago where the exhibit described a child born with spina bifida and hydrocephalus, and . . . asked people to vote on whether the child should live or die. I voted that the child should live, but when I voted, the child was losing by quite a few votes.

When these things happen, I get worried. I wonder if people are saying that they think the world would be a better place without me. I wonder if people just think the lives of people with disabilities are so full of misery and suffering that they think we would be better off dead. It's true that my life has suffering (especially when I'm having one of my eleven surgeries so far), but most of the time I am very happy and I like my life very much. My mom says she can't imagine the world without me, and she is convinced that everyone who has a chance to know me thinks that the world is a far better place because I'm in it. (18)

- Having a child with a serious disease or disorder does not necessarily cause an unhappy family life. In fact, such a child can enrich the life of the family. As one study group from the Hastings Center noted: "Families with children who are seriously ill or disabled often can find meaning and satisfaction in their lives, despite many obstacles. They are able to derive genuine joy from their children, as do other parents. They discover that their mutual commitment to the child has created an increased closeness among their members, 'involvement,' and personal growth. Siblings, by their own accounts, have become more sensitive and caring adults due to their experiences in helping to care for a seriously ill or disabled family member." (19)

Preimplantation Genetic Diagnosis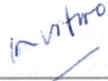

Rather than starting a pregnancy, undergoing prenatal diagnosis, and selectively aborting a fetus affected by a genetic disease (like cystic fibrosis), couples at risk of transmitting a genetic disease now have the option of using preimplantation genetic diagnosis. This procedure typically begins with creating embryos through in vitro fertilization. The fertilized ova are allowed to develop to about the eight cell stage, at which time a cell is removed for genetic analysis. If the developing embryo is found to be free of the genetic disease for which it is being tested, it will be transferred to a woman's body to try to achieve a pregnancy. However, if the embryo is found to be affected by the genetic disease, the embryo is not implanted. (15) Affected embryos are discarded. (20, 21)

Whether preimplantation genetic diagnosis is judged an ethically permissible course of action depends on how one answers the question of when human life first begins. If one believes that an embryo at the eight cell stage is not yet a human being, then one will not have any ethical qualms about disposing of the embryos affected by the genetic disease. On the other hand, if one believes that human life begins at conception/fertilization, one will see the disposal of the affected embryos as killing a human being and in the same category as abortion. (21)

Abortion in the Case of Rape

When a woman voluntarily engages in sexual relations knowing the risks of conceiving a child (and we know that no method of artificial contraception is one hundred percent safe), then it might be argued that she gives any child conceived the right to use her body. This simply does not apply, however, in the case of rape, where sex is forced upon a woman against her will. Some who are generally against abortion are still willing to allow it in those rare cases in which conception occurs as the result of rape. Thus, abortion in the case of rape deserves special attention.

It is generally accepted that there can be morally legitimate cases of killing in self-defense. Some argue that a woman who has been raped is simply defending herself against the attack in having an abortion. (22) However, those totally opposed to abortion might claim that the self-defense justification for killing is being incorrectly applied here. First of all, they might point out that the rapist, not the fetus, is the aggressor against whom the woman may take protective action. Further, there is a sense in which the fetus too is a victim of the rapist, in that the fetus was conceived in circumstances in which it was not wanted.

No one denies that it is traumatic and very difficult for a woman who is pregnant as a result of rape to carry the fetus to term. Nevertheless, in this situation an opponent of abortion from the Christian religious tradition might appeal to the New Testament parable of the Good Samaritan:

> A man was going down from Jerusalem to Jericho, when he fell into the hands of robbers. They stripped him of his clothes, beat him and went away, leaving him half dead. A priest happened to be going down the same road, and when he saw the man, he passed by on the other side. So too, a Levite, when he came to the place and saw him, passed by on the other side. But a Samaritan, as he traveled, came where the man was; and when he saw him, he took pity on him. He went to him and bandaged his wounds, pouring on oil and wine. Then he put the man

on his own donkey, took him to an inn and took care of him. The next day he took out two silver coins, and gave them to the innkeeper. "Look after him," he said, "and when I return, I will reimburse you for any extra expense you may have."

"Which of these three do you think was a neighbor to the man who fell into the hands of robbers?"

The expert in the law replied, "The one who had mercy on him."

Jesus told him, "Go and do likewise." (Luke 10: 30-37)

The point of this story is that the "Good Samaritan went out of his way, at some cost to himself, to help one in need of it." (22) Philosophical ethicists might call this an *act of supererogation:* an act which is morally commendable but which no one can be expected or obliged to perform. Similarly, it might be categorized as an act of supererogation for a woman who has been raped to carry the fetus to term in order to give the child life. (22) However, working within a religious framework, a woman might be strongly encouraged to go beyond what is strictly required and refrain from having an abortion.

CHAPTER SUMMARY

Key Terms and Concepts

abortion: the termination of a pregnancy with resulting death of the human fetus.

spontaneous abortion: a miscarriage; the termination of a pregnancy caused by purely natural factors.

induced or procured abortion: the termination of a pregnancy caused by human action.

indirect abortion: one type of induced/procured abortion occurring when the direct, immediate purpose of a procedure is to treat the mother for a threatening pathology, but the death of the fetus is also an inevitable result.

direct abortion: one type of induced/procured abortion occurring when the direct, immediate purpose of the procedure is to destroy the human fetus or to expel it when it is not viable. The term "abortion" as commonly used refers to direct abortion.

Key Points

- Three different positions have been taken on the moral permissibility of abortion: a) abortion on demand; that is, the view that abortion is permissible at any time during a pregnancy for any reason whatever; b) the view that abortion is permissible in a limited number of cases (for example, rape, incest, when the pregnancy threatens the well-being of the mother); and c) the view that abortion is never permissible.
- Abortion is commonly debated in terms of rights possessed by the mother and by the fetus respectively. In support of abortion, the following claims are made:
    - A woman has a right to a normal sex life, and is entitled to use abortion when artificial contraception fails.
    - A woman has a right to control what happens to her body.
- In opposition to abortion, the following claims about rights are made:
    - When a woman voluntarily engages in sexual relations, she gives any child who may be conceived the right to use her body.
    - The fetus's right to life takes precedence over hardships which may be experienced by the mother due to pregnancy and/or caregiving responsibilities for a child.
- One very common argument against abortion is that it is the killing of an innocent human being. This argument assumes that the embryo/fetus is a human being.
- Exactly when human life begins remains a matter of controversy.
- A utilitarian line of argument to justify aborting abnormal fetuses is that abortion will prevent suffering for both the family and the child and that it will benefit society by saving resources.
- Those opposed to aborting abnormal fetuses make the following points:
    - Families having a child with a serious disease can still have a happy and satisfying family life.
    - A child with a serious disease can still have abilities that enable the child to enjoy a good quality of life.
    - With some diseases, the severity of the symptoms varies from individual to individual, so that one could abort a child who would only be mildly affected.
    - A disease is not the totality of the person; persons suffering from diseases can make positive contributions to society through abilities they possess.
- The ethical permissibility of preimplantation genetic diagnosis, as involving the discarding of embryos, depends on one's view of whether the early embryo is a human being.

- Some who are generally against abortion consider it permissible in the case of rape. Abortion in this case is defended on grounds of self-defense. However, there are also people who encourage women who have been raped to make the sacrifice of carrying the pregnancy to term in order to give the child the gift of life.

FOR FURTHER DISCUSSION

1. Abortion is a very controversial issue. This chapter has set out the arguments both for and against the moral permissibility of abortion in various cases. Looking at these arguments, which of the following positions do you personally adopt on the abortion issue?
    - abortion on demand (that is, abortion is permissible at any time during a pregnancy for any reason);
    - abortion is permissible only in certain cases (specify which ones);
    - abortion is never permissible.

    What reasons can you give to defend the position you take?
2. Divide the class into groups representing the three positions listed in (1) above. Then have a formal debate about the positions.
3. This chapter has set out the reasons for citing various times during embryonic and fetal development as the beginning of human life. Looking at the evidence, at what time do you personally think that human life begins? What reasons are persuasive to you?

References

1. Benedict M. Ashley, O.P. & Kevin D. O'Rourke, O.P., *Health Care Ethics: A Theological Analysis*, 4th ed. (Washington, DC: Georgetown University Press, 1997).
2. Judith Jarvis Thompson, "A Defense of Abortion," *Philosophy and Public Affairs* 1/1 (Fall 1971): 47-66.
3. Mary Anne Warren, "On the Moral and Legal Status of Abortion," *Monist* 57/1 (January 1973): 43-61.
4. *Roe v. Wade* 410 United States Reports 113; decided January 22, 1973.
5. Daniel Callahan, "How Technology Is Reframing the Abortion Debate," *Hastings Center Report* (February 1986), p. 34.

6. John T. Noonan, Jr., "An Almost Absolute Value in History," in John T. Noonan, Jr. (ed.), *The Morality of Abortion: Legal and Historical Perspectives* (Cambridge, MA: Harvard, 1970).
7. Ronald Munson, *Intervention and Reflection Basic Issues in Medical Ethics*, 8th ed. (Belmont, CA: Thomson Wadsworth, 2008).
8. Robert P. George and Christopher Tollefsen, *Embryo A Defense of Human Life* (New York: Doubleday, 2008).
9. "Concepts of Death" in Rem B. Edwards and Glenn C. Graber (eds.), *Bioethics* (San Diego: Harcourt Brace Jovanovich, 1988).
10. Andre E. Hellegers, "Fetal Development," *Theological Studies* 31/1 (March 1970): 3-9.
11. Ronald M. Green, *The Human Embryo Research Debates* (New York: Oxford University Press, 2001).
12. Tom L. Beauchamp and LeRoy Walters, *Contemporary Issues in Bioethics*, 6th ed. (Belmont, CA: Thomson Wadsworth, 2003).
13. Leon R. Kass, "Implications of Prenatal Diagnosis for the Human Right to Life" in Bruce Hilton, Daniel Callahan, Maureen Harris, Peter Condliffe & Burton Berkeley (eds.), *Ethical Issues in Human Genetics: Genetic Counseling and the Use of Genetic Knowledge* (New York: Plenum, 1973).
14. Edmund N. Santurri, "Prenatal Diagnosis: Some Moral Considerations" in Edward D. Schneider (ed.), *Questions about the Beginning of Life* (Minneapolis: Augsburg, 1985).
15. Ricki Lewis, *Human Genetics*, 5th ed. (New York: McGraw-Hill, 2003).
16. Panel on cystic fibrosis, College Course 25, "Ethical, Legal, and Social Implications of the Human Genome Project," Dartmouth College, July 2, 1997.
17. Lecture by Adrienne Asch, College Course 25, "Ethical, Legal and Social Implications of the Human Genome Project," Dartmouth College, July 10, 1997.
18. Ricki Lewis, *Human Genetics Concepts and Applications*, 2nd ed. (Dubuque, IA: Wm. C. Brown, 1997).
19. Arthur Caplan and Cynthia B. Cohen (eds.), "Imperiled Newborns," Hastings Center Project Report, *Hastings Center Report* 17/6 (December 1987): 5-31.
20. Human Fertilisation and Embryology Authority and Advisory Committee on Genetic Testing, *Consultation Document on Preimplantation Genetic Diagnosis*. http://www.hfea.gov.uk/cps/rdc/xbcr/hfea/ PGD document.pdf. Accessed March 2009.

21. Vatican Congregation for the Doctrine of the Faith, *Dignitas Personae* (2008). http://www.usccb.org/comm/Dignitaspersonae/Dignitas_Personae.pdf. Accessed March 2009.
22. Jane English, "Abortion and the Concept of a Person," *Canadian Journal of Philosophy* 5/2 (October 1975): 233-43.

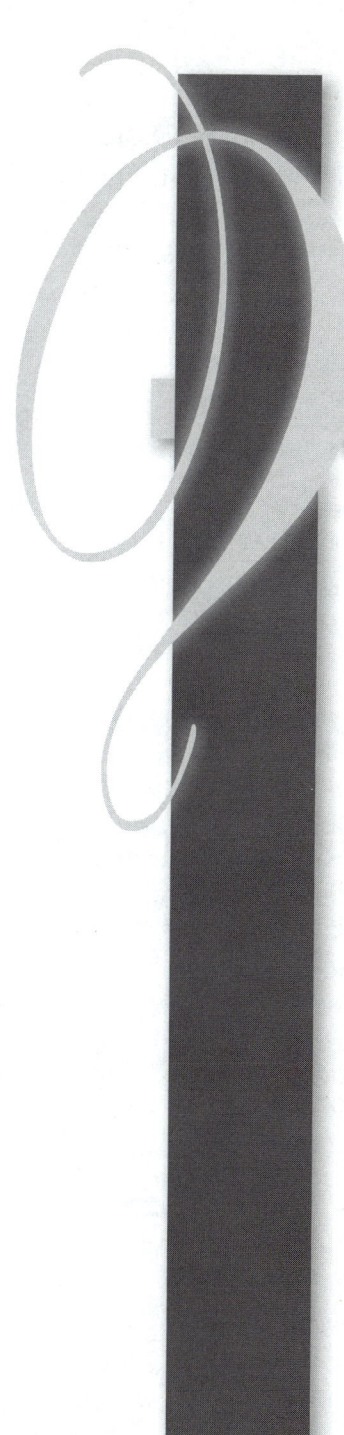

Chapter 4

Assisted Reproductive Technologies

The way we can go about having children has been dramatically changed by the development of assisted reproductive technologies (ART) such as artificial insemination, surrogate motherhood, in vitro fertilization, and the use of donor sperm and ova. First and foremost, these technologies are intended to assist married couples overcome problems of infertility. However, the use of these technologies can be extended to enable single persons and same-sex couples to have children. These technologies can also assist couples trying to avoid transmission of a genetically based disease to their children.

When one sees the happiness of people who have a child when they thought they could never have one at all, it seems one can only express gratitude for the technologies that make this possible. Nevertheless, some have voiced concerns about these technologies from an ethical point of view.

Chapter Four

In this chapter you will learn about:

- ethical issues that have been raised about such assisted reproductive technologies as artificial insemination by donor, surrogate motherhood, and in vitro fertilization;
- how concerns about assisted reproductive technologies interface with ethical theories.

Case Study

Ellen Peterson has just completed her educational training as a clinical laboratory technologist. One of her professors has recommended her for a job at a nearby university fertility clinic, and she has been called to come for a job interview.

As part of the interview process, Ellen meets with the clinic's director. She finds the director tremendously enthusiastic about the kind of work being done at the clinic to help infertile couples realize their dream of having a child. The director tells her the story of one couple who had recently used the clinic's services.

"The couple had married in their late twenties, after completing graduate school," he stated. "After trying unsuccessfully to become pregnant for two years, the wife decided to see a doctor who is a fertility specialist for a work-up. No problems were detected. She then convinced her husband to see the doctor. Testing indicated that her husband is infertile. His sperm count is extremely low, and the doctor did not think that even "pooling sperm" would work to enable the conception of a child—collecting and storing his sperm so that the total sperm count is higher when injected into his wife. However, the doctor told them not to lose hope in their dream of having a family, and referred them to our fertility clinic to explore the technologies currently available to assist infertile couples in having children. The couple came to our clinic and decided to use the procedure of artificial insemination by donor (AID). A pregnancy was achieved using AID. Just this morning the couple visited our clinic to show off their new baby daughter and to thank our staff for their help!"

Ellen can appreciate the joy the clinic's work has brought to this couple by enabling them to have a much wanted child. At the same time, Ellen herself comes from a religious background that considers the use of donor sperm equivalent to an act of adultery. Before she accepts a position at this clinic, she wants some time to reflect on the ethics of the procedures the clinic is performing.

■ ■ ■

Artificial Insemination by Donor

Artificial insemination (AI) is a fertilization procedure in which a fine catheter (tube) is used to deposit sperm into a woman's cervix (intracervical insemination—ICI) or into her uterus (intrauterine insemination—IUI). The sperm may come either from the woman's husband (AIH) or from a donor (AID). (1, 2)

Artificial insemination by donor may be sought by a married couple "if the male partner suffers from severe sperm problems (extremely low count, no motile sperm, no sperm with normal morphology, sperm without the ability to penetrate the egg or the complete absence of sperm)." (3) This would include men suffering from infertility due to radiation or chemotherapy treatment for cancer, congenital problems, spinal cord injuries, sexually transmitted diseases and infections such as gonorrhea, and vasectomies that cannot be successfully reversed. (4) Thus this procedure has sometimes been referred to as *therapeutic donor insemination (TDI)*. (3, 5) Or again, a couple may seek AID for genetic reasons; for example, when the husband is the carrier of a dominant gene for a genetic disorder or when both husband and wife are carriers of a recessive gene for a genetic disorder. (4)

In the case study Ellen Peterson alludes to one ethical concern that has been expressed about AID in the case of a heterosexual married couple: it involves going outside the bond of the marriage to have a child. Some see it as part of the very meaning of marriage that the spouses pledge to have children only through each other. (6) Anecdotal evidence indicates that *feelings of infidelity* can accompany the use of AID by married couples:

> A couple who had been treated for male infertility for three years had just finished their second and last IVF cycle in which they did not get fertilization. . . . They made an appointment with the psychologist to discuss donor insemination. The husband stated that he was ready to move on to DI [donor insemination]. . . . His wife was far more hesitant, telling the psychologist timidly, "I've never told anyone this, but my husband is the only man I have ever had sex with. I'm afraid that having another man's sperm inside me would make me feel like I was sleeping with someone else."
> Men similarly may express feelings of hesitancy about DI due to fears that if their wife conceives, they will feel as if she is carrying another man's child. (4)

The same ethical concern about breaking the marital covenant would apply to any technology involving the use of donor sperm or ova by a heterosexual married couple.

Another ethical issue pertains to the sperm donor himself. Someone can donate blood, and then just walk away. But donating semen seems different. It has more significant consequences: a new human life is produced through artificial insemination. Thus the question has been raised of whether, from an ethical point of view, a sperm donor has any responsibilities to the child produced using his sperm, and if so, how this impacts the individuals who are raising his biological child. (7)

One approach to ethics—utilitarianism—makes judgments of rightness and wrongness based on the consequences of a course of action for everyone affected (see chapter 1). On the one hand, AID is seen as having benefits (good consequences) for a couple in comparison with adoption. Specifically, both the husband and wife can be involved in the pregnancy from conception onward, sharing the experience of delivery and the early days of the baby's life. The desire on the part of the mother to carry a child is satisfied as it cannot be in adoption. Further, the husband and wife can exercise control over the child's prenatal care and need not worry that something in the prenatal environment may cause problems later in the child's life. Moreover, there is a greater chance that the child's physical appearance will at least match that of the mother and, if there are several children, they are more likely to resemble one another. There also need be no subconscious fear of the sudden appearance of the natural mother, as there may be in adoption. Finally, AID affords privacy to a couple while adoption is a public statement about their infertility. (4, 8, 9)

On the other hand, there can be negative psychological consequences for a couple using AID. A Canadian study of 120 couples using AID indicated that use of this procedure "generates intense and troublesome feelings both within and between spouses." (4) The researchers found that "common reactions for men are loss of self-esteem, emotional withdrawal, and temporary impotence." (4) For their part, women experience "anger, guilt, and a wish to make reparations." (4)

Moreover, AID carries the negative consequence of a loss of genetic continuity. While most children "have some qualities of each parent that are recognizable," couples considering the use of AID "must face their feelings of sadness about not being able to see some of the father's traits reflected in their children." (4) Further, couples who have a strong sense of family roots may feel that donor insemination is severing their ancestral ties and that they may disappoint their families by choosing AID. They may also worry that, if their family learns about their use of AID, the grandchild will not be loved or accepted in the same way a biological child would be. (4)

AID may also have some negative consequences for the child. If the sperm donor is anonymous, lack of knowledge of the child's paternal heritage may prove harmful if the child should need a reliable family medical history. (10)

Further, with the practice of anonymous donation comes the possibility of sibling marriages. (10)

There can likewise be negative ramifications for the sperm donor and those with whom he is in relationship. A sperm donor must face the fact that "he will have offspring whom he will not know." (4) Further, "if the donor has children of his own, they will have half-siblings whom they do not know," and the donor "must think about whether he would tell his children about their unknown genetic siblings." (4) A sperm donor must also "consider whether he will tell his spouse (or future spouse) and how his spouse might react to the information." (4)

In sum, a utilitarian in ethics would weigh both the positive and negative consequences for the whole range of affected persons in making a judgment about the rightness or wrongness of AID (see chapter 1).

It is noteworthy that AID has been used as part of a eugenic program to produce superior human beings. One such program was the Repository for Germinal Choice in San Marcos, California, whose donors of germinal material consisted of Nobel Laureates in science and other high achievers. The recipients were young women selected for their superior health and intellect, under 35 years of age, with sterile husbands who agreed to the use of AID. The aim of the project was to increase the number of offspring of the most creative scientists of our time. (11) In a similar vein, the Fairfax Cryobank in Fairfax, Virginia, has a special (and more expensive) category of sperm donors called "Fairfax Doctorate," consisting of "donors who are in the process of earning, or have completed, a Doctorate degree." (12) These individuals include "medical, dental, chiropractic, law (Juris doctorate), veterinary, optometry, pharmacy, and Ph.D. students and graduates." (12)

Our case study and discussion of it have focused on the use of AID by heterosexual married couples. However, some single women and lesbian couples have used AID in order to bear a child. (13) In conjunction with surrogate motherhood, AID can also be used by single men to have a child.

Case Study

Jerry Zellner has worked in the laboratory of the Wentworth Fertility Clinic for the past five years. Recently the clinic's director asked him to serve on a special committee to deal with a problem situation.

Once the legal arrangements have been made with an attorney, the clinic has been providing artificial insemination services for women who have agreed to be surrogate mothers. At the first committee meeting, Gerald learns about the problem that brought about the formation of the committee. A surrogate mother who had been inseminated at the clinic recently gave birth to twins. The couple who contracted with the surrogate is refusing to take two babies. They claim they legally agreed to have only one child, and they have already picked out the one they want. The surrogate is married with two sons of her own, and decided to work as a surrogate mother to earn some extra money for her own family. Financially, she can't possibly assume care of yet another child.

The committee must make recommendations concerning the fate of the two babies. If the contracting couple succeeds in their claim to assume care of only one of the babies, who should decide which one they get? Does the surrogate have any responsibilities for the second child as the biological mother? Should arrangements be made to put the second child up for adoption?

Apart from these immediate concerns, one committee member suggests that the clinic undertake a comprehensive study of its services to surrogate mothers to prevent problems for the clinic in the future. Jerry concurs with this suggestion, commenting that the study should address the ethical dimensions of surrogacy as well as clinical and legal issues. He has come to wonder if we as a society need to be more selective in our use of reproductive technologies. Perhaps some technologies are okay morally, but others are not.

■ ■ ■

Surrogacy

Surrogate motherhood can take different forms. In one case, a couple contracts with a woman who is artificially inseminated with the husband's sperm and who carries the pregnancy with a pledge to give the child to the contracting couple once it is born. Because the surrogate contributes her ovum to the conception of the child, she is genetically related to the child. In gestational surrogacy, on the other hand, ova and sperm are fertilized in vitro (IVF) and then developing embryos are implanted in the uterus of a woman who carries the pregnancy with the intent of giving the child to another couple once it is born. The ova used in the IVF procedure can be provided either by the woman who is to raise the child (contracting couple) or by a donor. Often a surrogate is a stranger contracted through an agency. She receives a substantial monetary fee for her services. Sometimes a relative or friend will serve as a surrogate in an informal, noncommercial relationship. (10, 14)

Surrogacy can be attractive to a couple with infertility problems because it is a quicker procedure than legal adoption and because, when artificial insemination is used, it gives the couple a child who is at least partly related to them genetically. (10) Some have pointed out a biblical precedent for surrogate motherhood in the case of Abram and Sarai. Since Sarai was herself infertile, she made arrangements for Abram to have a child with her Egyptian maid Hagar (Genesis 16:1-4). (11)

Surrogacy is clearly an issue of particular concern to women. Feminists have been split in their assessment of surrogacy. Some have defended the practice on the grounds that women should be allowed to control their own bodies, with surrogacy being one of their reproductive choices. (15) Other feminists have opposed surrogacy, and for a variety of reasons. For one thing, it is seen as an affront to the dignity of women: "When a woman provides womb service, the feminist issue surfaces. Women object to being baby factories or sex objects because it offends their human dignity."(15) Indeed, surrogate motherhood has been compared to prostitution. (15) Surrogacy also involves the potential for psychological harm to women since it requires suppression of the natural bonding between mother and child. It can be emotionally traumatic for a woman to surrender the child she has carried. (16, 17) This has been especially evident when surrogate mothers have engaged in legal custody battles to keep the children they have carried. (10) Furthermore, the monetary payment that often accompanies surrogacy carries the danger of exploiting women who are poor. Such monetary compensation can put pressure on poor women to use their bodies to support themselves and their families. (18) It is feared that "it is always going to be poor women who have the babies and rich women who get them." (15)

Feminists have had long-standing concern for the welfare of children, and it has been argued that surrogacy arrangements involve potential harm to children. Parents may expect more of a child for whom they have paid $10,000. (16) A child produced through a surrogacy arrangement may be deprived of important medical information about his or her heritage. (18) Especially when the surrogate mother is a stranger hired through an agency, the practice of surrogate motherhood increases the possibility of half-sibling marriages occurring. (18) Further, should the child produced in a surrogate arrangement turn out to be mentally impaired or physically handicapped, the fate of the child can be in question. Who will want the child? Will the child end up in a state institution? (19)

Some women who have served as surrogate mothers have themselves been married with children of their own. These children too may be harmed by surrogacy arrangements. Some of these children "have reported their fears that they may be sold like their half-brother or half-sister, and express a sense of loss at being deprived of a sibling." (17) In fact, it has been argued that "the widespread acceptance of commercial surrogacy would psychologically threaten all children."(17) This is because "it would change the way children are valued by people (parents and surrogate brokers)—from being loved by their parents and respected by others, to being sometimes used as objects of commercial profit-making." (17)

In sum, Jerry Zellner in our case study is entirely correct in thinking that, apart from any legal considerations, there are ethical issues to consider about surrogacy. Concerns about the impact of surrogacy on the women serving as surrogates can be connected with Kant's ethics. (See chapter 1.) Does surrogacy simply "use" women to produce children for others and fail to respect the intrinsic worth of the surrogates themselves? Concerns about potential harm for children resulting from the practice of surrogacy are reinforced by the ethical principle of nonmaleficence. (See chapter 1.)

Case Study

Chuck Forbes works as a physician assistant at a fertility clinic which is part of a university hospital and medical school. He sometimes conducts the initial interview with couples coming to the clinic for the first time.

Today Chuck has an interview with Rita and John Linden. Rita and John are now in their mid-thirties. When they got married after college they decided to postpone having children until they both got established in their careers and had achieved some degree of financial security. Four years ago they decided they were ready to start a family, but their efforts to conceive a child never resulted in a pregnancy. It was discovered that Rita had blocked fallopian tubes which prevented ova from reaching her uterus. She underwent surgical repair of her oviducts, but still could not conceive. The Lindens' physician has suggested they go to the fertility clinic to investigate in vitro fertilization (IVF).

Rita and John consider themselves to be "pro-life." They have heard concerns expressed by their friends about the fate of embryos in the IVF process. They tell Chuck Forbes that they want to be fully informed about the IVF procedure before they make a decision to go this route to try to have a child.

■ ■ ■

In Vitro Fertilization

In vitro fertilization (IVF) involves stimulating multiple ova to develop, retrieving them from the woman, fertilizing them in the laboratory with sperm, and transferring resulting embryos to a woman's body to attempt to achieve a pregnancy. (20) The ova and sperm used in the IVF process can either come from a married couple, or one or both can be donated.

Multifetal pregnancies (twins, triplets, or more) can result if too many embryos are transferred to a woman at a given time. Thus the number of embryos transferred is determined by the quality of the embryos and by weighing the risks for a multifetal pregnancy against the risk of failing to conceive since, as female age increases, the implantation rate of embryos tends to decline. (20) Embryos not immediately transferred to a woman are typically frozen for later use. (10)

There is concern that IVF poses physical risks to the children conceived through this technology:

> A study published in the *New England Journal of Medicine* in 2002 found that babies conceived by IVF techniques and intracytoplasmic sperm injection . . . have an 8.6% risk of such birth defects as heart abnormalities, cleft palate, and undescended testicles; the usual risk is 4.2%. A second study in the same journal found that babies conceived through reproductive technologies have 2.6 times the usual risk of low birth weight, which is associated with heart and lung problems and poor cognitive development. (10)

Further studies found that such assisted reproductive technologies carry an increased chance of Beckwith-Wiedemann syndrome, a condition involving enlarged organs and childhood cancer, and of retinoblastoma, a cancerous eye tumor. (10) Ethically, the principle of nonmaleficence directs us to avoid taking actions that bring harm to others. (See chapter 1.)

In the case study, Rita and John Linden express concern about the fate of the embryos created in the IVF process. Embryonic loss does occur with IVF. It is known that not all the embryos transferred to a woman will implant to achieve a viable pregnancy. (20) Further, frozen embryos can become "spare" if a couple does not want to use them for further attempts to achieve a pregnancy. Such excess embryos can be donated to infertile couples. (21) However, such excess embryos can also be discarded or donated for scientific research (22), such as embryonic stem cell research which involves destruction of the embryo. (See chapter 18.) Whether actions which involve the loss, discarding, or destruction of human embryos are ethically problematic depends on one's view of the status of the early stage embryo. (See chapter 3.)

Some are also concerned that technological methods of reproduction, such as IVF, which separate the conception of a child from an interpersonal act of sexual intercourse and make it into a purely laboratory procedure, will create a mentality of viewing children as "commodities to be manufactured." As stated by one couple who tried such technological methods:

> Paul Lauritzen, speaking for himself and his wife, sums up the experience of their efforts to generate children through technological processes by saying: "The process of reproduction in a clinical environment (causes) a way of thinking of ourselves and our world in terms that are incompatible with intimacy . . . once procreation is separated from sexual intercourse, it is difficult not to treat the process of procreation as the *production of an object to which one has the right as a producer.*" (23; italics added)

A mentality of treating our children as "objects" would violate Kantian ethics. (See chapter 1.)

Further, there is concern that the use of donor sperm or ova with IVF and other reproductive technologies can lead to disruption and confusion of parent-child and family relationships. Scenarios such as the following are not far-fetched. Suppose that Sally, a woman in her mid-forties who is divorced, decides to remarry and that she and her new husband (who is a childless widower) want to start a family. Sally is now infertile, and consultation with an IVF clinic indicates that she is not a suitable candidate for that procedure. However, the clinic does tell the couple that the husband's sperm could be used to fertilize a donor egg, and that the embryo could be implanted in a surrogate mother who would carry the child to term for them. Sally has a daughter in her twenties from her previous marriage, and the daughter offers to donate the ovum to be used in the IVF procedure so that the child will be genetically related to Sally. Thus Sally will be in the unusual position of being both mother (in terms of social relationships) and grandmother (biologically) to the child, and Sally's daughter will be both the child's mother (biologically) and its sister (in terms of social relationships). (24)

In the future, a child could have three sets of parents. The child could be conceived in vitro from ova and sperm coming from a man and woman who may be either living or dead (frozen sperm or ova). A surrogate mother could carry the child to term, and then surrender the child to yet another couple to raise him or her. In other words, reproductive technologies have the potential to separate *biological* parenting from *gestational* parenting from *social* parenting. (25) What will this kind of separation do to a child psychologically? And to the child's sense of personal identity?

CHAPTER SUMMARY

Key Terms and Concepts

assisted reproductive technologies (ART): medical technologies aimed at helping people have children.

artificial insemination (AI): a fertilization procedure in which a fine catheter (tube) is used to deposit sperm into a woman's cervix (intracervical insemination—ICI) or into her uterus (intrauterine insemination—**ICI**). The sperm may come either from the woman's husband (**AIH**) or from a donor (**AID**).

surrogacy/surrogate motherhood: a reproductive arrangement in which a woman carries a pregnancy with the intent of giving the child, once it is born, to another with whom she has contracted. The pregnancy may be achieved either through artificial insemination with the contracting man's sperm, or by implantation of embryos after in vitro fertilization (**gestational surrogacy**).

in vitro fertilization (IVF): a procedure that involves stimulating multiple ova to develop, retrieving them from the woman, fertilizing them in the laboratory with sperm, and transferring resulting embryos to a woman's body to attempt to achieve a pregnancy.

Key Points

- Assisted reproductive technologies have the benefit of enabling people to have a child when they thought they could never have one at all because of problems with infertility. At the same time, ethical concerns have been expressed by some about these technologies.
- While artificial insemination by donor has advantages over adoption, it can also have negative repercussions for the couple using it, the child conceived through this procedure, and the sperm donor himself.
- The use of donor gametes (sperm or ova) by a married couple means going outside their marriage to have a child, and raises the question of breaking their marital covenant to each other.

- The practice of surrogate motherhood has raised concerns about the treatment and exploitation of women.
- Surrogate motherhood can also have negative consequences for the child produced through this arrangement and for the surrogate mother's own children.
- In vitro fertilization and the concomitant freezing of embryos ultimately bring about the loss, discarding, and destruction of embryos. Whether such actions are judged ethically permissible depends on one's view of the status of the early human embryo.
- There is some evidence of IVF causing an increased incidence of birth defects. There is likewise concern that in vitro fertilization (and other reproductive technologies) will create a mentality of viewing children as commodities as well as lead to disruption and confusion of the parent-child relationship.

FOR FURTHER DISCUSSION

1. Sarah and John Goldberg were married three months ago. Through a program at their synagogue they have learned that they belong to a population at risk for Tay-Sachs disease. An infant with this genetic disease appears to develop normally for the first few months of life. Then, as his/her nerve cells become distended with fatty material, a progressive mental and physical deterioration occurs. The child becomes blind, deaf, and unable to swallow, and muscles begin to atrophy with paralysis setting in. There is currently no cure for Tay-Sachs and, even with the best of care, children with this disease usually die by age 4. (26)

    Tay-Sachs is a recessive inherited genetic disorder, so that a person must have two copies of the gene to have the disease. Someone can be a "carrier," having just one copy of the gene; in this case, the person will be unaffected by the disease. Both parents must be carriers of the gene for Tay-Sachs in order for a child to be affected by this disease. If both parents are carriers, there is a 25 percent chance for any pregnancy that the child will be affected by Tay-Sachs. (26)

    While Sarah and John dream of having several children, they definitely don't want any child of theirs to be afflicted with such a devastating disease as Tay-Sachs. For this reason they decide to undergo the simple blood test that will determine if they are carriers. The worst case scenario occurs. They find out that they are both carriers for Tay-Sachs.

Unwilling to give up their dream of having children, Sarah and John make an appointment with a genetic counselor. The counselor tells them that they have the following options for having children:

1. Take a chance and conceive a child naturally, but with the intent of accepting the child whatever his/her health condition.
2. Conceive a child naturally but use prenatal diagnosis to determine the genetic status of the fetus, with the intent of aborting any fetus affected by Tay-Sachs. (See chapter 3.)
3. Use in vitro fertilization to produce embryos which will undergo preimplantation genetic diagnosis, using only those embryos not affected by Tay-Sachs to try to achieve a pregnancy. (See chapter 3.)
4. Use donor sperm or ova from someone who does not carry the gene for Tay-Sachs to conceive a child through artificial insemination or in vitro fertilization.
5. Forgo having their own biological children and adopt.

- *Reflecting critically on the material presented in this chapter (and the chapter on abortion), which course(s) of action do you regard as **ethically permissible**? What reasons can you give to support your judgment? If you consider a particular course of action to be ethically permissible, can you answer any ethical concerns that might be voiced about it?*
- *From practical and ethical points of view, which do you think is the **best** course of action for Sarah and John to take? Why?*

2. In the second case study in this chapter, a special committee at the Wentworth Fertility Clinic must deal with a situation in which a surrogate mother has unexpectedly given birth to twins and the contracting couple is unwilling to accept two children. From an ethical point of view, what duties and responsibilities apply to this situation? What recommendations should the committee make regarding the fate of the two babies?
3. In the second case study, the Wentworth Fertility Clinic is planning to undertake a comprehensive study of its services to surrogate mothers. Suppose you are an employee of the clinic who is asked to serve on this study committee. Would you argue for or against the clinic continuing to provide surrogacy services? What is the rationale for your position?
4. The case studies in this chapter have focused on heterosexual married couples using assisted reproductive technologies. Do you think there are any additional ethical issues involved with reproductive clinics making their services available to women and men who are single but want to have a child? To same-sex couples?

References

1. MedicineNet.com, *MedTerms Medical Dictionary*. http://www.medterms.com. Accessed March 2009.
2. DocShop.com, *Artificial Insemination*. http://www.docshop.com/education/fertility/treatments/artificial-insemination. Accessed March 2009.
3. Infertility, Gynecology, & Obstetrics (IGO) Medical Group of San Diego, The Fertility Institute, "Therapeutic Anonymous Donor Insemination." http://www.igomed.com/fertilityserv.htm. Accessed 2002.
4. Susan Lewis Cooper and Ellen Sarasohn Glazer, *Choosing Assisted Reproduction Social, Emotional & Ethical Considerations* (Indianapolis, IN: Perspectives Press, 1998), pp. 157-8.
5. Infertility and IVF Center, St. Louis, MO, "Artificial Insemination." http://www.ivfctrstl.org/ai-meanings.htm. Accessed 2002.
6. See, for example, Pope Pius XII, "Christian Norms of Morality" in Kevin D. O'Rourke, OP & Philip Boyle, OP, *Medical Ethics: Sources of Catholic Teachings* (St. Louis: Catholic Health Association, 1989).
7. Ronald Munson, "Artificial Insemination and Donor Responsibility" in Ronald Munson (ed.), *Intervention and Reflection Basic Issues in Medical Ethics*, 4th ed. (Belmont, CA: Wadsworth, 1992).
8. Edward D. Schneider, "Artificial Insemination" in Edward D. Schneider (ed.), Questions About the Beginning of Life (Minneapolis: Augsburg, 1985).
9. International Federation of Fertility Societies, "International Consensus on Assisted Procreation," Artificial Insemination with Donor Sperm. http://www.mnet.fr/iffs/a_artbis.htm. Accessed 2002.
10. Ronald Munson, "Reproductive Control" in Ronald Munson (ed.), *Intervention and Reflection Basic Issues in Medical Ethics*, 8th ed. (Belmont, CA: Thomson Wadsworth, 2008).
11. D. Gareth Jones, *Brave New People* (Grand Rapids, MI: Eerdmans, 1985).
12. Fairfax Cryobank, "About our Donors." http://www.fairfaxcryobank.com/aboutdonors.shtml. Accessed March 2009.
13. Reproductive Technologies Inc., The Sperm Bank of California. http://www.thespermbankofcalifornia.com. Accessed March 2009.
14. Conceptual Options A Center for Surrogacy and Egg Donation. http://www.Surrogacy-EggDonation.com. Accessed March 2009.
15. Ruth Macklin, "Is There Anything Wrong with Surrogate Motherhood? An Ethical Analysis," *Law, Medicine & Health Care* 16/ 1-2 (Spring/Summer 1988): 57-64.

16. Lori B. Andrews, "Surrogate Motherhood: The Challenge for Feminists," *Law, Medicine & Health Care* 16/1-2 (Spring/Summer 1988): 72-80.
17. Elizabeth S. Anderson, "Is Woman's Labor a Commodity?" *Philosophy and Public Affairs* 19/1 (Winter 1990).
18. Herbert T. Krimmel, "The Case against Surrogate Parenting," *Hastings Center Report* 13/5 (October 1983): 35-9.
19. Ronald Munson, "Reproductive Control" in Ronald Munson (ed.), *Intervention and Reflection Basic Issues in Medical Ethics*, 5th ed. (Belmont, CA: Wadsworth, 1996).
20. Advanced Fertility Center of Chicago, In Vitro Fertilization (IVF). http://www.advancedfertility.com. Accessed March 2009.
21. See, for example, the "Snowflake" adoption program of Nightlight Christian Adoptions. http://www.nightlight.org/snowflakeadoption.htm. Accessed March 2009.
22. Genetics and IVF Institute, "Fertility Services." http://www.givf.com. Accessed March 2009.
23. Jean deBlois, SCJ, Patrick Norris, OP, & Kevin O'Rourke, OP, *A Primer for Health Care Ethics Essays for a Pluralistic Society* (Washington, DC: Georgetown University Press, 1994).
24. "When Baby's Mother Is Also Grandma—And Sister," *Hastings Center Report* 15/5 (October 1985): 29.
25. Arthur L. Caplan, "The Ethics of In Vitro Fertilization" in Richard T. Hull (ed.), *Ethical Issues in the New Reproductive Technologies* (Belmont, CA: Wadsworth, 1990).
26. National Institute of Neurological Disorders and Stroke of the National Institutes of Health, *NINDS Tay-Sachs Disease Information Page*. http://www.ninds.nih.gov/disorders/taysachs/taysachs.htm. Accessed March 2009.

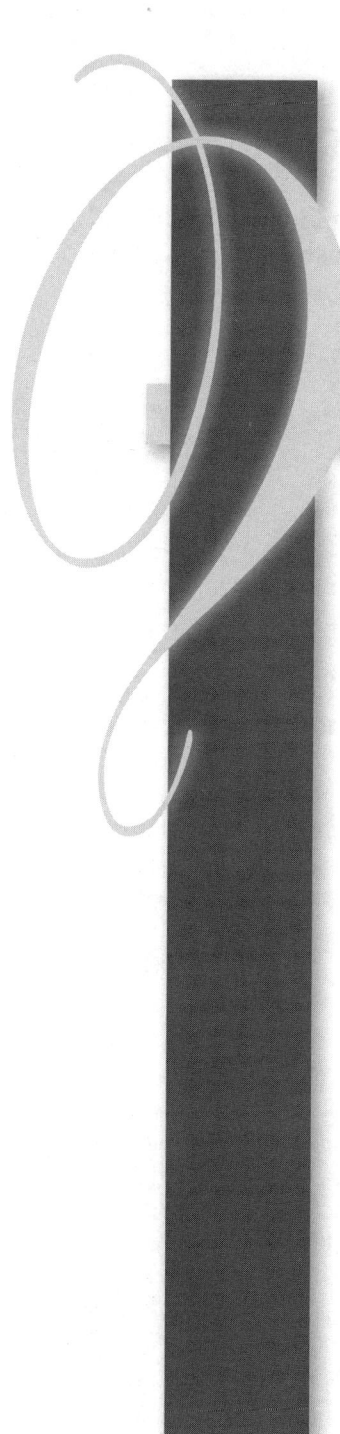

Chapter 5

Treatment Decisions for Seriously Ill Newborns

When parents await the birth of a child, what they have in mind is the birth of a normal, healthy child who is "cute and cuddly." But sometimes parents undergo the emotional trauma of having a child who has serious health problems. Infants can be born prematurely and with low birth weight. These infants can have problems with immature lung development, feeding, susceptibility to infections, internal hemorrhage, and anemia. (1) Some infants are born with life-threatening congenital abnormalities. Examples are anencephaly, a condition in which the cerebral cortex of the brain is absent; spina bifida, which involves an opening in the spine; and Down syndrome, a condition involving mental retardation that may be accompanied by a gastrointestinal blockage. (1) In such cases, decisions must often be made whether to give medical treatments to the infant or withhold them.

Chapter Five

In this chapter you will learn about:

- ethical principles for making decisions about giving or withholding medical treatments in the case of seriously ill newborns;
- the scope of parental rights in treatment decision making for their children;
- the pros and cons of practicing euthanasia in the case of seriously ill newborns.

Case Studies

Emilio Sanchez is a laboratory technician at a university medical center. Emilio usually does the lab work for the neonatal unit, and he knows the physicians and nursing staff in that unit quite well. During the last week there have been two especially difficult cases in that unit that have left Emilio wondering about the right thing to do for seriously ill newborns.

On Monday, Charles and Marilyn Birmingham had a son with anencephaly, a neural tube defect resulting in absence of a major portion of the brain (forebrain and cerebral cortex). A baby born with anencephaly is usually blind and deaf, unconscious, and unable to feel pain. There is no cure or standard treatment for anencephaly, and the prognosis for babies born with this condition is extremely poor. If the infant is not stillborn, the infant usually dies within a few hours or days after birth. (2) After prenatal testing, the Birmingham's pediatrician had told them that their baby would be born with this condition, but they decided to carry the pregnancy to term anyway. In fact, Charles and Marilyn made it clear that, if the baby were born alive, they wanted the child placed in the neonatal intensive care unit and "everything possible done" to save the child's life. Their pediatrician had reluctantly agreed to their request. However, the nurses in the neonatal intensive care unit were very uncomfortable with this decision and felt that they were being asked to prolong the suffering of the child. They felt relieved when the child died a day and a half after birth.

The stress level for staff increased when Sarah Gordon gave birth to a baby girl with Down syndrome and, along with this, a digestive system blockage which prevents normal intake of food and liquids. Sarah's pediatrician assured her that the blockage could be surgically corrected and the sooner, the better. However, Sarah indicated that she wanted to allow the child to die. "My husband is unemployed and I am a student at a community

> college, and we're trying to get our own lives together," she stated. "We just couldn't deal with a special needs child. My parents live in another state and my husband's parents both have health problems, so they are not able to help us with caregiving. Besides, the intestinal blockage is nature's way of saying that the baby shouldn't live. She'll be better off in heaven." The staff in the neonatal unit disagreed with the mother's decision and discussed whether they should seek a court appointed guardian for the baby girl to authorize the surgery. When Emilio Sanchez hears about this, he wonders, as an outsider, if they would be violating Sarah's rights as a parent in taking this course of action.

■ ■ ■

The Challenges of Caring for a Child with a Serious Illness or Disability

In the second case, Sarah Gordon feels overwhelmed by the prospect of taking care of a child with special needs. The hardships involved with raising a seriously ill or disabled child have been described at some length by a Hastings Center study group on imperiled newborns:

> . . . families may experience stress of different kinds when responsible for the care of a child with serious illness or disabilities. . . . Apart from concerns about finances, the greatest single source of stress that they describe is the responsibility for home health care. When some parents have attempted to provide intensive care at home for their infants in need of dialysis or ventilator support, they have found this too stressful to continue. Parents who have not had the responsibility of providing such intensive care also report that the demands on their energy and inner resources are high, and that some of them experience "burn-out" over an extended period of time. Fatigue is a major problem for families whose children require constant care.
>
> Families also describe stress created by their fears about an uncertain future. Their anxiety is generated not only by the ambiguity that surrounds their child's future development and needs, but also by their concern about whether adequate services will be available for them at later points in time. They face the possibility that they will have a lifetime

of extensive and unassisted responsibility for their child that will not taper off as the child grows older. A related source of stress for families is their feeling of social isolation and stigma. Researchers have found, for instance, that 74 percent of parents of children who are severely developmentally disabled have neighbors who object to having their child associate with the disabled child. In 40 percent of these families, parents are never able to go out together; one always has to be home to care for the child. . . .

> They report that their experiences of fatigue, loss of free time, marital tension, anger, depression, guilt, and a sense of helplessness and isolation tend to wear them down. Some experience a "chronic sorrow" that they cannot overcome. There are some reports of a higher rate of child abuse and marital breakup in families with children who are seriously ill or disabled. The contemporary realities of shifting employment currents, new roles for men and women, and rapid mobility can make a positive parental response to children who need extensive care difficult to sustain, for careers are attenuated and movement to suit employment limited. The reverse is also true in that parents who have wishes to remain at home to care for their children have been forced into the workplace in order to meet the expenses of their child's treatments." (3)

However, some would point out that these hardships are not the whole story. Assistance is available to help parents and families cope with these difficulties. On a financial level, governmental assistance may be available to help with the cost of care. (4) On an emotional level, "individual and group counseling can substantially alleviate anxiety, guilt, and frustration, and enable parents to cope with underlying conflicts triggered by the birth and the adaptation required." (4) Perhaps even more importantly, it has been pointed out that the experience of caring for a seriously ill or handicapped child can have a positive aspect to it:

> Finally, in many cases, the experience of living through a crisis is a deepening and enriching one, accelerating personality maturation, and giving a new sensitivity to the needs of spouse, siblings, and others. As one parent of a defective child states: "In the last months I have come closer to people and can understand them more. I have met them more deeply. I did not know there were so many people with troubles in the world." (4)

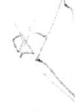
In sum, some would argue that "although we must recognize the burdens and frustrations of raising a defective infant, it does not necessarily follow that these costs require nontreatment."(4)

To ensure that the rights of seriously ill or disabled children are not compromised, some have recommended that treatment decisions for seriously ill newborns should focus almost exclusively on the welfare of the child himself. For example, the Council on Ethical and Judicial Affairs of the American Medical Association has taken the position that "the primary consideration for decisions regarding life-sustaining treatment for seriously ill newborns should be what is best for the newborn." (5) Similarly, the President's Commission for the Study of Ethical Problems in Medicine and Biomedical and Behavioral Research recommended that "parents should be able to choose among alternative treatments with similarly beneficial results and among providers, but not to reject treatment that is reliably expected to benefit a seriously ill newborn substantially...." (1) Because "it is all too easy to undervalue the lives of handicapped infants," the Commission "excludes consideration of the negative effects of an impaired child's life on other persons, including parents, siblings, and society." (1)

Standards for Treatment Decision Making

Chapter 6, "Decisions about Using or Forgoing Life-Sustaining Treatments," will present the *principle of weighing benefits and burdens*, a widely accepted principle for making such decisions. This chapter will discuss other standards that have been proposed by ethicists specifically for the case of seriously ill newborns. These standards reflect the focus on the infant himself or herself. We will present three different standards developed by ethicists.

Medical Indications Policy   This standard focuses exclusively on the physical condition of the child. It directs that if a treatment is available that will work medically, it should be provided to the child. No infant should be denied medical treatments simply on the basis of his or her handicap or future quality of life. Treatment should be provided to all infants except when the infant is in the process of dying or when the treatment itself is medically inadvisable. (3)

Best Interest of the Child   This standard allows the child's quality of life to be taken into account. It directs that an infant should be treated except when the infant is dying, or when the treatment itself is medically inadvisable, or when continued life would be worse for the child than an early death. (3)

Relational Potential Standard   This standard is based on the belief that "the meaning, substance, and consummation of life is found in human relationships." (6) According to this standard, it is permissible to withhold medical treatments from an infant when the infant's potential for engaging in human relationships is simply nonexistent, or would be utterly submerged and undeveloped in the mere struggle to survive. (6)

How do these standards apply to our case studies? First, how do these standards apply to the case of the Birmingham's anencephalic son? According to the medical indications policy, it would be permissible to forgo all life-sustaining treatments for the baby once it is born since the child can be regarded as in the process of dying; the prognosis for babies born with anencephaly is extremely poor, with such babies typically dying within a few hours or days after birth. The best interests standard also allows treatment to be forgone when an infant is dying. Similarly, the relational potential standard would justify withholding treatment from an anencephalic infant, although on different grounds: the absence of a cerebral cortex (the part of the brain primarily responsible for the psychological functions of consciousness, thought, and feeling) makes the child incapable of entering into characteristically human interrelationships. (6) In sum, according to each of these principles, it is ethically justifiable to forgo life-sustaining treatments for the Birmingham's anencephalic son, as the nurses in the neonatal intensive care unit believe is best.

However, the case of Sarah Gordon's daughter with Down syndrome and a digestive system blockage is different from an ethical point of view. According to the medical indications policy, the fact the child has the handicap of Down syndrome and will not have a "normal life" is irrelevant to making the treatment decision. What should be considered are her physical condition (digestive system blockage) and whether there is a medical treatment available for this condition. The blockage is indeed a *treatable* condition through surgery; it is not the case that the child is in an irreversible process of dying. Further, the surgical repair of the digestive system blockage is medically advisable; in fact, the doctor thinks that the sooner the surgery is performed, the better. Therefore, according to the medical indications policy, Sarah's daughter should have this treatment.

The standard of the best interest of the child would consider all these factors, but would go beyond the requirements of the medical indications policy in also taking into account the child's quality of life. Here is one description of the life of Down syndrome children:

> Developmental milestones (such as sitting, standing, and walking) come slowly, and toilet training may take several years. People with Down syndrome tend to have warm, loving personalities and enjoy art and music. Intelligence varies greatly, from those with profound mental retardation, to those who can follow simple directions, read, and use a computer. One young man with Down syndrome graduated from a junior college and another starred in a television series. (7)

At the present time, the degree of mental retardation that Sarah's daughter will suffer is not clear. This is one of the special challenges of making medical treatment decisions for newborns—the long-range outcome may be ambiguous or uncertain. (1, 3) There is a real chance, however, that Sarah's daughter can have a quality of life that will make continued existence preferable to death. Thus, Sarah's daughter is not disqualified from receiving treatment according to the standard of the best interest of the child. This standard does not justify Sarah's decision to withhold the surgery from her daughter.

The relational potential standard for medical treatment decision making is different from the other two standards in making primary the ability of the child to enter into characteristically human relationships. By this standard, it is legitimate to withhold medical treatment under either of two conditions: (a) the child simply will not have the capability of entering into human relationships; (b) so much time and effort would have to be devoted to mere physical survival that the child could not really cultivate human relationships. The description of Down syndrome children indicates that many can enter into characteristically human relationships. They have "warm, loving personalities." They can share art and music with other people. They can participate in society by holding certain levels of jobs. Only if a Down syndrome child suffered from very severe mental retardation or had some other severe physical problem might it be questionable that the child could pass the relational potential standard for receiving medical treatment. In the case of Sarah's daughter, the digestive system blockage can be surgically repaired. The degree of mental retardation she will suffer is not clear at this point. Thus, Sarah's daughter is not disqualified from receiving medical treatment using the relational potential standard. Again, this standard does not justify withholding the surgery to correct the digestive system blockage.

Which of these three standards ought to be adopted as the principle for making medical treatment decisions in the case of seriously ill newborns? The answer may depend in part on one's conception of the purpose of health care and on other values one holds. Is the purpose of health care merely to address physical needs, or to address physical needs as a means of enabling a person to achieve a certain level of function and quality of life? Is existence and life on the physical plane intrinsically valuable? Or is such existence valuable only as enabling a person to engage in certain sorts of activities? And if we take into account quality of life considerations in making decisions about giving or forgoing medical treatments for newborns, can we ever get beyond such judgments being subjective and reflective of personal biases?

Who Should Make the Treatment Decision?

In the second case, the nurses in the neonatal unit disagree with Sarah Gordon's decision to deny surgery for her infant daughter. They are contemplating going to court to get someone appointed as the baby's legal guardian who will authorize the surgery to be performed. Emilio Sanchez, the laboratory technician for the neonatal unit, wonders whether they would be violating Sarah's rights as a parent in taking this course of action.

Ethically and legally, there is a presumption in favor of parental decision-making authority in the case of seriously ill newborns:

> The ethical basis for according parents primary authority over decisions concerning medical care is rooted in the strong ties of affection and concern that parents have for their offspring. The love that parents have for their children is the basis for the belief that parents will endeavor to formulate decisions about medical care in accordance with their child's best interest. Indeed, under ordinary circumstances, there seems to be no one else who could make better decisions for children than their parents, for no one else is as familiar with their needs or as likely to cherish them.
>
> . . . The law justifies this assignment of decision making authority to parents . . . because parents necessarily must play an ongoing role in governing the lives of their children. The law recognizes that parents, to be parents, must be accorded the right to make basic decisions as to the welfare of their children. (3)

At the same time, "parents may be reeling emotionally from the shock of having a seriously ill child instead of the normal, healthy infant they had imagined." (1) They may be poorly informed about the child's medical condition and long-term prognosis. (1) In these situations health care providers can serve as advisors to parents, helping them "in sorting through possible treatment options and their consequences." (3)

Ideally, treatment decisions should be made jointly by parents and health care providers, and agreed upon by both. Nevertheless, cases may arise where parents reject treatment for a child that health care providers view as clearly effective, or insist on treatment that health care providers see as futile or harmful. (3) In such situations, health care staff may call upon the resources of an ethics committee or an infant care review committee to assist in resolving the conflict. (5; see chapter 2)

Should an ethics consult not succeed in reconciling the views of parents and health care providers, legal recourse is available. As persons unable to protect themselves, infants fall under the *parens patriae* power of the government. (1) In the exercise of this power, the state can override parental decisions to ensure that the child is not neglected or abused. The state's perceptions of what is in the interests of the child can take precedence over the views and decisions of parents. (1)

In the case of Sarah Gordon and her daughter, the hospital nurses see Sarah as acting against her daughter's interests in denying her the surgery that would allow normal intake of food and liquids. Legally, they can go to court to try to override Sarah's decision.

In sum, while there is a presumption in favor of parental decision-making authority in the case of seriously ill newborns, it is also recognized that particular parents may not make reasonable decisions, and that parental authority over their children is not absolute.

Euthanasia in the Case of Seriously Ill Newborns

Thus far we have focused on the issue of forgoing life-sustaining treatments for seriously ill newborns. Some would go even farther and allow euthanasia for (at least some) seriously ill newborns. If abortion is permitted, why draw the line at birth for the permissibility of killing? After all, newborns seem closer to unborn fetuses than to adults. (3) Moreover, once a decision is made not to use life-sustaining treatments, an earlier death through euthanasia may mean less suffering for the infant since sometimes an infant does not die immediately when life support is withdrawn or withheld. (3)

For example, infants falling into the following category have been proposed as candidates for euthanasia:

> Finally, there are infants with a hopeless prognosis who experience what parents and medical experts deem to be unbearable suffering. Although it is difficult to define in the abstract, this group includes patients who are not dependent on intensive medical treatment but for whom a very poor quality of life, associated with sustained suffering, is predicted. For example, a child with the most serious form of spina bifida will have an extremely poor quality of life, even after many operations. This group also includes infants who have survived thanks to intensive care but for whom it becomes clear after intensive treatment has been completed that the quality of life will be very poor and for whom there is no hope of improvement. (8)

Named after a university medical center in the Netherlands, the *Groningen Protocol* would allow euthanasia of such infants when five criteria are met:

- The infant's diagnosis and prognosis must be certain.
- The infant must be experiencing hopeless and unbearable suffering.
- At least one independent physician must confirm that the first two conditions are met.
- Both parents must give their informed consent.
- The termination procedure must be performed in accord with the accepted medical standard. (9)

Needless to say, the concept of euthanasia for seriously ill infants has proven very controversial.

The Hastings Center study group on imperiled newborns raised several concerns about allowing infanticide as a matter of social policy. For one thing, health care professionals are fallible human beings, so that errors can occur in the prognosis given for a newborn and medical conditions can be misidentified. Further, if euthanasia were allowed for newborns, abuses could occur. Some parents could advocate killing their infants to serve their own purposes rather than their infants' welfare. Individual physicians may have strong feelings about particular kinds of disabilities being "worse than death" and so push the option of euthanasia. Hospitals may see opportunities to cut cost through the practice of euthanasia. (3) Moreover, in response to the argument that dying infants will suffer in the absence of euthanasia, it can be pointed out that "advances in pain management make it possible to relieve all or almost all pain." (3)

For these reasons, the Hastings Center study group recommended that social policy should *not* permit the active killing of seriously ill and disabled infants. (3)

CHAPTER SUMMARY

Key Terms and Concepts

medical indications policy: a principle specifically for treatment decision making in the case of seriously ill newborns that maintains that no infant should be denied medical treatments simply on the basis of his or her handicap or future quality of life. Treatment should be provided to all infants except when the infant is in the process of dying or when the treatment itself is medically inadvisable.

best interest of the child: a principle specifically for treatment decision making in the case of seriously ill newborns that maintains that infants should be treated except when the infant is dying, or when the treatment itself is medically inadvisable, or when continued life would be worse for the child than an early death.

relational potential standard: a principle specifically for treatment decision making in the case of seriously ill newborns that maintains the permissibility of withholding medical treatments from an infant when the infant's potential for engaging in human relationships is simply nonexistent or would be utterly submerged and undeveloped in the mere struggle to survive.

parens patriae power: a governmental power pertaining to persons who are unable to protect themselves, such as children, allowing the government to override parental decisions in order to ensure that the child is not neglected or abused.

Key Points

- There are hardships involved in caring for and raising a child with a serious illness or with disability. At the same time, assistance is available to parents and families to cope with these difficulties. There can be positive, enriching aspects to the experience of caring for a seriously ill or handicapped child.
- To safeguard the interests and rights of the child, decisions about medical treatment for seriously ill newborns should focus on the welfare of the child himself or herself.
- Several standards have been proposed for medical treatment decision making specifically in the case of seriously ill newborns: the medical indications policy, the best interest of the child, and the relational potential standard.
- There is a presumption in favor of parental decision-making authority in the case of seriously ill newborns. However, it is recognized that particular parents may not make reasonable decisions so that, legally, parental authority is not absolute. The court system has the power to override parental decisions to ensure that the child is not neglected or abused.
- Some argue for the practice of euthanasia in the case of seriously ill newborns as an extension of the legally accepted practice of abortion and in order to provide a quick end to the infant's suffering. Opponents of euthanasia are concerned about errors being made in the prognosis for an infant, and about possible abuses of the practice of euthanasia. In addition, it is pointed out that good pain management can relieve the suffering of seriously ill newborns as they die.

FOR FURTHER DISCUSSION

1. Has anyone in your family or someone else you know suffered from a disease or disability since birth? How do you see the quality and value of their lives? How do they assess the quality and value of their lives?
2. Three different principles were presented for making treatment decisions in the case of seriously ill newborns: the medical indications policy, the principle of the best interest of the child, and the relational potential standard. Which of these principles do you personally favor for use in making treatment decisions for seriously ill newborns? Why?
3. A policy statement on *Treatment Decisions for Seriously Ill Newborns* formulated by the Council on Ethical and Judicial Affairs of the American Medical Association includes the following directives:

   The primary consideration for decisions regarding life-sustaining treatment for seriously ill newborns should be what is best for the newborn. Factors that should be weighed are (1) the chance that the therapy will succeed, (2) the risks involved with treatment and nontreatment, (3) the degree to which the therapy, if successful, will extend life, (4) the pain and discomfort associated with the therapy, and (5) the anticipated quality of life for the newborn with and without treatment.
   Care must be taken to evaluate the newborn's expected quality of life from the child's perspective. Life-sustaining treatment may be withheld or withdrawn from a newborn when the pain and suffering expected to be endured by the child will overwhelm any potential joy during his or her life. When an infant suffers extreme neurological damage, and is consequently not capable of experiencing either suffering or joy, a decision may be made to withhold or withdraw life-sustaining treatment. When life-sustaining treatment is withheld or withdrawn, comfort care must not be discontinued. (5)

   - *Compare and contrast these directives with the principles presented in this chapter; namely, the medical indications policy, the principle of the best interest of the child, and the relational potential standard.*
   - *If these directives were used to guide the treatment decision in the case of the Birmingham's anencephalic son, what decision would be made?*
   - *If these directives were used to guide the treatment decision in the case of Sarah Gordon's daughter born with Down syndrome and a digestive system blockage, what decision would be made?*

4. The authors of the Groningen Protocol propose that infants suffering from the most serious form of spina bifida are candidates for euthanasia. (8) Do some background research on spina bifida. After learning the facts about spina bifida in its various forms, do you think that it is ever appropriate to forgo medical treatments for an infant suffering from spina bifida? Do you agree that infants suffering from the most serious form of spina bifida deserve euthanasia?

References

1. President's Commission for the Study of Ethical Problems in Medicine and Biomedical and Behavioral Research, *Deciding to Forego Life-Sustaining Treatment* (March 1983; reprint New York: Concern for Dying).
2. National Institute of Neurological Disorders and Stroke, *Anencephaly Information Page*, http://www.ninds.nih.gov/disorders/anencephaly/anencephaly.htm. Accessed March 2009.
3. Arthur Caplan and Cynthia B. Cohen (eds.), "Imperiled Newborns," Hastings Center Project Report, Hastings *Center Report* 17/6 (December 1987): 5-31.
4. John A. Robertson, "Involuntary Euthanasia of Defective Newborns: A Legal Analysis," *Stanford Law Review* 27 (1975): 246-61.
5. Council on Ethical and Judicial Affairs of the American Hospital Association, *Current Opinions* E-2.215. http://www.ama-assn.org/ama/pub/about-ama/our-people/ama-councils/council-ethical-judicial-affairs.shtml. Accessed March 2009.
6. Richard McCormick, S.J., "To Save or Let Die The Dilemma of Modern Medicine," *Journal of the American Medical Association* 229/2 (July 8, 1974): 172-76.
7. Ricki Lewis, *Human Genetics: Concepts and Applications*, 2nd ed. (Dubuque, IA: Wm. C. Brown, 1997).
8. Eduard Verhagen and Pieter J.J. Sauer, "The Groningen Protocol—Euthanasia in Severely Ill Newborns," *New England Journal of Medicine* 352/10 (March 10, 2005): 959-62.
9. James Lemuel Smith, "The Groningen Protocol: The Why and the What" in Ronald Munson, *Intervention and Reflection Basic Issues in Medical Ethics*, 8th ed. (Belmont, CA: Thomson Wadsworth, 2008).

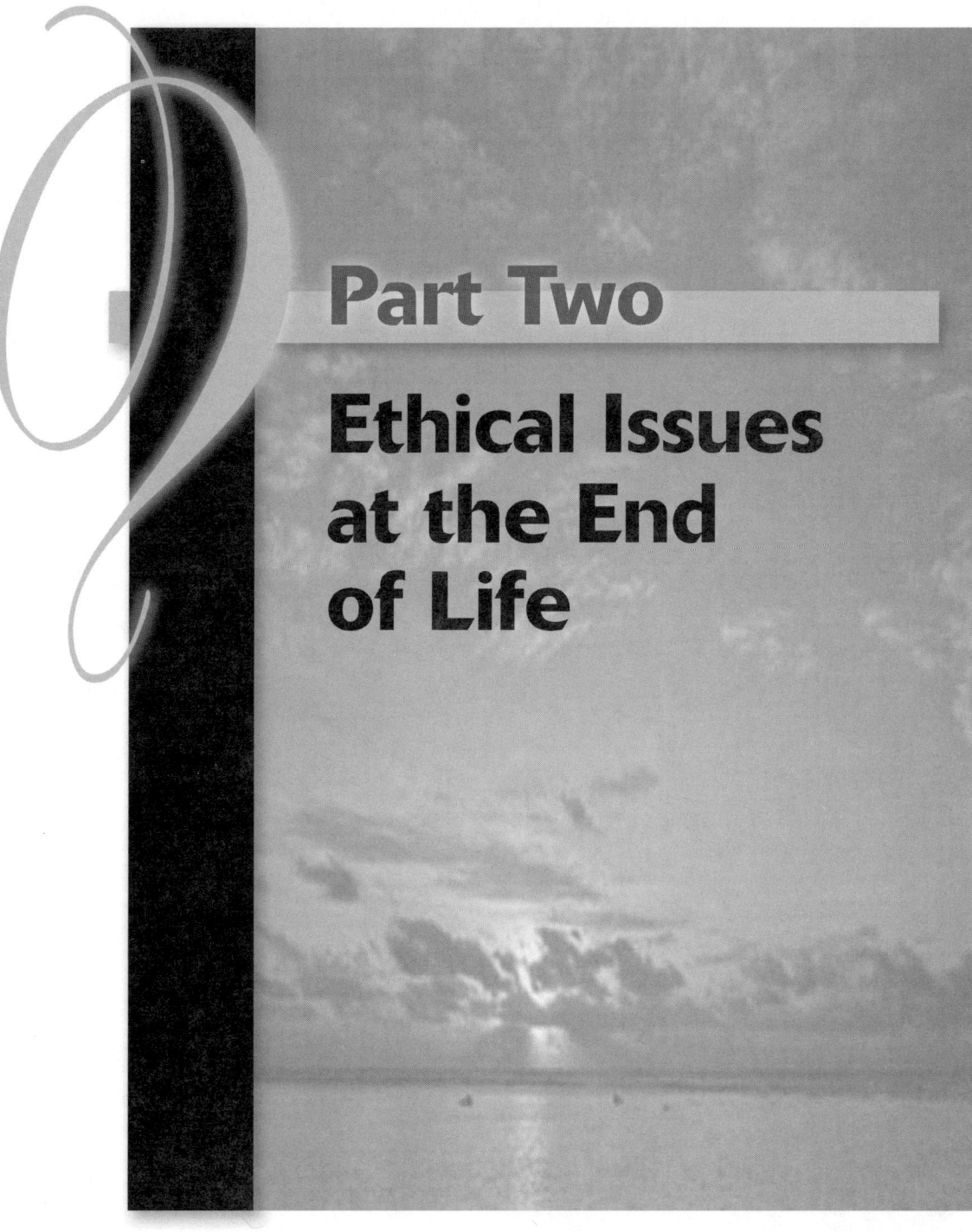

Part Two

Ethical Issues at the End of Life

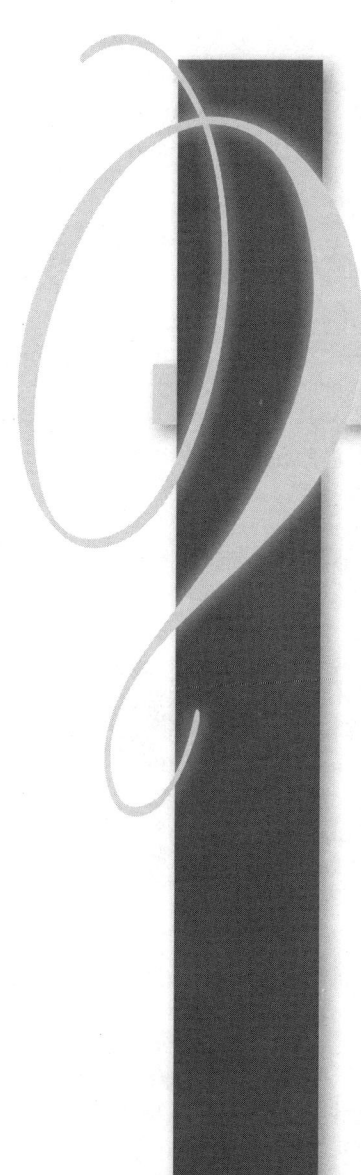

Chapter 6

Making Decisions about Using or Forgoing Life-Sustaining Treatments

A *life-sustaining treatment* is "any medical intervention, technology, procedure, or medication that is administered to a patient in order to forestall the moment of death, whether or not the treatment is intended to affect the underlying life-threatening disease(s) or biologic processes." (1) Examples of life-sustaining treatments include chemotherapy, kidney dialysis, resuscitation, the use of a ventilator, and tube feeding. The administration of antibiotics or blood pressure medication can also fall into this category in some cases.

In this chapter you will learn about:

- how to make decisions about using or forgoing life-sustaining treatments;

- whether it is permissible to withdraw a treatment once it has been started;
- the difference between forgoing a life-sustaining treatment and euthanasia;
- controversies concerning futile care.

Case Study

Roger and Kate Smith, both 76, have been residents of the Oak Park Home, a multi-level facility, for a year. Three years ago Roger had a cancerous tumor in his stomach, but chemotherapy had worked in shrinking it and causing the cancer to go into remission. However, within the last month the cancer has recurred.

Chemotherapy is promptly begun for Roger. However, Roger's doctor is honest with him that, this time around, the chemotherapy will probably slow the growth of the tumor and prolong his life but is not likely to "cure" his cancer as it did before.

The first time Ray had cancer, he had tolerated the chemotherapy treatments reasonably well. But this time he experiences nausea and vomiting, and feels so "washed out" for a week after each treatment that he cannot even enjoy his grandchildren when they come to visit him. In addition, the pain from the cancer is considerable.

To make things worse, two months later Roger develops pneumonia. Because of his overall weakened physical condition, Roger's physician recommends hospitalization with antibiotic treatment and placement on a ventilator with supplemental oxygen. Initially, Roger agrees.

However, after five days in the hospital Roger writes a note to his respiratory therapist, Sue Martin, indicating that he no longer wants these treatments for his pneumonia. In fact, he indicates to his wife and his physician that he wants to stop chemotherapy treatments as well. All these treatments, he feels, are only prolonging his suffering. He states that he has lived a full life, and is ready to die. Roger had been a very successful attorney, and no one doubts that he is still sharp mentally.

Roger's wife Kate is sometimes at the hospital when Sue Martin looks in on Roger. In conversations with Kate, Sue learns that Roger and Kate have three children and that two of the children support Roger's decision to forgo all medical treatments while his wife Kate and one of their daughters disagree. They feel that Roger has "given up too soon." After all, he beat the odds with cancer once before, and he has grandchildren to live for and enjoy.

> Sue knows that, if a decision is made to stop all medical treatments as Roger wishes, she will be involved in withdrawing the ventilator support. The conflict that exists within Roger's family makes Sue herself wonder what the right thing to do really is.
>
> ■ ■ ■

Ethical Principles for Making Decisions about Life-Sustaining Treatments

Two ethical principles are commonly brought into discussions about using or forgoing life-sustaining treatments: the *principle of autonomy* and the *principle of weighing benefits and burdens.*

Autonomy refers to self-determination, to directing the course of one's own life. Patient autonomy entails that a competent patient has a right to be involved in decision making about medical treatments, and indeed, to make the final decision about using or forgoing treatments (see chapter 1).

In the case of Roger Smith, there is no doubt that he is "still sharp mentally" and thus competent to make medical treatment decisions. Roger has clearly expressed his desire to stop all the medical treatments being administered. According to the principle of autonomy, Roger's health care providers should agree to Ralph's wishes and stop the administration of antibiotics, the use of a ventilator, and chemotherapy treatments.

Sometimes the principle of patient autonomy is presented in such a way that health care providers are expected to abide by the wishes of the patient no matter what he wants and no matter what the rationale for his decision. Experience with putting the principle of autonomy into practice is causing us to recognize certain limitations to patient choices. One of these limitations is the expectation that patients should make their treatment decisions in accord with accepted principles of health care ethics.

Historically, a distinction was made between *ordinary* and *extraordinary* medical treatments. The accompanying moral principle stated that ordinary treatments must always be provided when needed but there is no obligation to use treatments that are extraordinary. (3) Aspirin, blood pressure medication, and antibiotics might be considered ordinary treatments. Ventilators, chemotherapy, and kidney dialysis might be given as examples of extraordinary treatments.

However, ethicists came to see problems with this distinction and the accompanying moral principle. Recently, ethicists have refined it into a *principle of weighing benefits and burdens*. This is not a completely new standard. Rather, it is an attempt to introduce clarity and precision into discussions by focusing on one of the traditional interpretations of the ordinary/extraordinary treatment distinction. (2, 3)

The principle of weighing benefits and burdens sets out the following criteria for making decisions about using or forgoing life-sustaining treatments:

- If a treatment provides more benefits than burdens from the patient's perspective, the treatment should be provided.
- If the burdens of a treatment outweigh its benefits from the patient's perspective, it is permissible to forgo (i.e., withhold or withdraw) the treatment.
- If it is unclear whether the burdens or benefits are greater, it is appropriate to err on the side of life and provide the treatment.
- If a treatment is useless or futile, not providing benefit to the patient, it is permissible to forgo (i.e., withhold or withdraw) the treatment. (1, 2, 3)

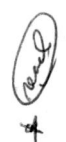

The first two criteria are something like a cost/benefit analysis. What are the benefits the treatment might bring? Will it bring about a cure (or even a partial cure) for the patient? Will it give the patient relief from pain? Will it increase the patient's physical mobility? Will it restore the patient's consciousness? Will it enhance the patient's ability to communicate with family and friends? On the other hand, are some aspects of the proposed treatment burdensome? Will the treatment itself cause the patient pain or substantial discomfort? Will the treatment entail any psychological burdens, such as depression? Will the patient have difficulty getting access to the treatment? (For example, will the patient have to drive a substantial distance each week to get the treatment?) Will the patient have to be restrained to tolerate the treatment? (For example, will the patient have to be restrained to prevent him from pulling out a feeding tube?) Will the treatment impose a financial burden on the patient or his family?

Balancing the sides, are the benefits of the treatment greater than the burdens? If the answer is yes, then the treatment should be undertaken. On the other hand, are the burdens greater than the benefits? Then it is morally permissible to forgo the treatment. Since individual patients may evaluate the benefits and burdens of a treatment differently, promoting the patient's good entails that benefits and burdens should be assessed *from the perspective of the particular patient*. (1)

It should be noted that our interpretation of the principle of weighing benefits and burdens includes benefits and burdens both for the patient (e.g., increasing the patient's physical mobility) and for other people (e.g., the cost of the treatment for the patient's family). It also includes benefits and burdens of both a purely medical nature (e.g., pain and discomfort caused by the treatment) and a non-medical nature (e.g., the cost of treatment). What is more controversial is the inclusion of quality of life considerations. Should we limit ourselves to consideration of the burdensomeness *of the treatment itself,* or should we consider the burdensomeness *of the life sustained* through a treatment? (2) For example, pneumonia was at one time called "the old person's friend" because it could bring about death for persons suffering from other debilitating diseases.

In some cases a treatment simply will not work physically for a patient. For example, some patients cannot tolerate tube feeding because the fluid would be too much for a weakened heart. (4) Or again, antibiotics are ineffective against viral (vs. bacterial) pneumonia. (5) In such cases, the treatment provides no benefit whatever to the patient. The principle of weighing benefits and burdens recognizes that when a treatment is useless or futile, there is no moral obligation to use it.

When using the principle of weighing benefits and burdens to make decisions about life-sustaining treatments, decisions are made on a case-by-case basis. There is no treatment which must automatically be used. Likewise, there is no treatment which can automatically be forgone. The question to ask is: What will this treatment do for this particular patient who is in this particular condition? Even if a treatment is commonly available (such as antibiotics), there is not necessarily a moral obligation to use it. (1)

In discussing life-sustaining treatments, we have spoken of both the principle of patient autonomy and the principle of weighing benefits and burdens. Is there a way of putting them together? While we should abide by the wishes of the patient, it is also true that patients should not make their decisions in a purely arbitrary way. We should encourage them and help them to look at the relative benefits and burdens of the treatment, and to make their decision on that basis.

How does all of this apply to the case of Roger Smith? First, do the benefits and burdens of the chemotherapy justify stopping this treatment? The chemotherapy is not expected to cure Roger's cancer. It is expected to slow the growth of the tumor and hence to prolong Roger's life, although we do not know for how long a time. Thus, while there is some benefit to Roger from the chemotherapy, the benefit is limited. On the other hand, the chemotherapy has some definitely burdensome aspects to it. Roger is experiencing nausea and vomiting from the chemotherapy, and treatments leave him feeling so "washed out" for a whole week that he cannot even enjoy his grandchildren when they come to visit him. Further, the pain Roger is experiencing from the cancer is considerable, and prolonging his life through administration of chemotherapy is only prolonging his pain. In addition, there are the costs of continued aggressive treatment to consider, not only the chemotherapy treatments themselves but the fact that Roger must be placed in a unit of the Oak Park Home which provides a higher level of nursing care and hence is more expensive. Roger may worry about what will happen to his wife Kate if their financial resources are depleted. In sum, in this case it would be reasonable to judge that the burdens of Roger's chemotherapy treatments outweigh the benefits, and thus stopping the chemotherapy treatments is a morally permissible course of action.

What about discontinuing the antibiotics for Roger's pneumonia and removing the ventilator support? This decision is more complex. The administration of antibiotics for pneumonia in itself may not be particularly burdensome. However, Roger views treating his pneumonia as prolonging his battle with cancer and the suffering of his dying process, and hence the treatment could be regarded as creating burdens in this respect. It is important to recognize that antibiotics can serve a dual role. Antibiotics can be life prolonging, but they can also be a form of palliative care providing comfort to the patient. Similarly, a ventilator can be a form of palliative care in providing oxygen support for comfort, and this is very different from prolonged respiratory support by ventilator. (6) If the antibiotics and ventilator are comfort measures for Roger, they are beneficial for him and thus might be continued until the pneumonia is cleared although the chemotherapy is stopped.

Misconceptions about Forgoing Life-Sustaining Treatments

The case of Roger Smith involves stopping chemotherapy. In the past, some have made a distinction between *withholding* a life-sustaining treatment (that is, never starting a treatment) and *withdrawing* a treatment (that is, stopping a treatment). Some judged that it is morally permissible to withhold a treatment but that, once started, a treatment cannot be stopped. (1) This kind of thinking has changed. Ethically, it is now considered just as permissible to withdraw a treatment as never to start it. (1)

Why has this change in attitude taken place? In some cases we may not be sure, in advance of using a life-sustaining treatment, whether it will benefit the patient or not. If we have the mentality "once a treatment is started, it cannot be stopped," we may be afraid of ever trying the treatment. This is because we would not want to be locked into a treatment that will not help the patient but will only prolong his dying process and suffering. Suppose we adopt a policy across the board of forgoing a treatment when its benefits are uncertain. This might mean that there are patients who would have benefited from the treatment who will never receive it and whose lives will be lost. Thus, time-limited trials of life-sustaining treatments are recommended. If it is unclear whether a treatment will benefit a patient, it should be tried out for a predetermined period of time and its effect evaluated. If it proves not to work physically or to be more burdensome than beneficial to the patient, then it should be withdrawn. (1)

It may be more difficult emotionally and psychologically for family members or health care workers to stop a treatment than never to start it. But if we have tried a treatment and then decide to withdraw it for lack of beneficial results, we can at least feel that we have done everything we can to help the patient. (1)

Some family members or health care workers may feel guilty about withdrawing a life-sustaining treatment. The reason is that they feel they will be doing something to cause the death of the patient. In other words, they are afraid that, in stopping a life-sustaining treatment, they will be engaging in an act of euthanasia. This fear is unfounded. Daniel Callahan clearly distinguishes euthanasia ("killing") from forgoing a life-sustaining treatment ("letting die") in terms of what is the *cause of death* and in terms of the *intention* behind the action:

> . . . as a reality of nature, killing and letting die are causally different. "Letting die" is only physically possible if there is some underlying disease that will serve as the cause of death. Put me on a respirator now, when I am in good health, and nothing whatever will happen if it is turned off. I cannot be "allowed to die" by having a respirator turned off if I have healthy lungs. It is wholly different, however, if a doctor gives me a muscle-relaxing injection that will paralyze my lungs. Healthy or not, those lungs will cease to function and I will die. That is what it means to "kill" someone as distinguished from "letting someone die." Put more formally, there must be an underlying fatal pathology if allowing to die is even possible. Nothing but the action of the doctor giving the lethal injection is necessary to bring about death.
>
> . . . Here is Rachels' second mistake: to assume that the intention in letting die is ordinarily the same as in killing, that is, to make a person dead. It is certainly the case that we *might* intend someone's death and turn off a machine to bring that about. But it is equally the case, and far more common in ordinary medical practice, that patients are allowed to die because of a judgment that it no longer makes sense, medically or morally or both, to continue life-extending treatment. Doctors have long stopped treating patients when their skills and art run out. There is no reason to think that, as a rule, it is because their intentional goal is to make people die. (7)

In sum, in the case of forgoing a life-sustaining treatment, there is an underlying fatal pathology which made the use of the life-sustaining treatment necessary in the first place and which will be the direct cause of the patient's death when the treatment is stopped. Further, the intent in withdrawing a life-sustaining treatment is not to destroy the patient, but to stop a treatment that is no longer justified medically or morally.

Another misconception about decisions to forgo life-sustaining treatment is that, once such a decision has been made, the patient will simply be abandoned by health care providers. This is not true. Pain medication and comfort care will still be provided. A slogan has surfaced in health care, "Care, not cure." (8) A time may come in a patient's illness when nothing more can be done medically to help the patient recover from the disease. At this stage the emphasis changes to one of relieving the symptoms of the disease and of enabling the patient to spend his final days in as comfortable and meaningful a way as possible.

Finally, if a decision has been made to stop treatment, this does not mean that the treatment must be withdrawn immediately. Time can be provided for family members and friends to say final good-byes and for religious rituals to take place before the treatment is stopped and the patient is allowed to die.

Case Study

Elaine Manion, 28, has been battling cystic fibrosis (CF) since birth. In spite of the daily therapy needed to clear her lungs, she has tried to stay active and live as normal a life as possible. She has become the manager of a restaurant, and teaches religious education classes to children in her church. Elaine knows that people with CF have a shortened life span, and that she is nearing the maximum life expectancy for persons with CF.

As Elaine nears her twenty-ninth birthday, her health begins to fail. She is repeatedly hospitalized. For several years Elaine has been working closely with Michael Adams, a respiratory therapist, and Jane Finnegan, a physical therapist who provides postural drainage therapy. Both Michael and Jane recognize that Elaine has begun the "final downhill slide."

During her latest hospitalization, Elaine's doctor, Marilyn Lee, advises her to have a Do-Not-Resuscitate (DNR) order. A cardiopulmonary arrest, Dr. Lee says, would simply be a part of her body giving out in the dying process. CPR might not work at all in restoring her heart beat and respiration and, even if it did, Elaine would likely suffer another arrest in a few days.

> Elaine, however, refuses to consent to a DNR order. She believes that God can work miracles for those who believe in him. In Elaine's view, deciding to forgo resuscitation—just standing by and allowing death to come—would show a lack of faith in God's power to heal. Elaine repeatedly tells Dr. Lee and her therapists that she wants all available treatments, including resuscitation.
>
> Dr. Lee feels strongly that resuscitation would be "futile" in Elaine's case. She is tempted to simply write a DNR order on Elaine's chart. This is a case, she believes, in which "the doctor knows best" and the patient is acting irrationally. Michael Adams agrees with Dr. Lee, but Jane Finnegan isn't so sure. After all, shouldn't health care providers first and foremost respect a patient's wishes?
>
> ■ ■ ■

The Question of Medical Futility

According to the principle of weighing benefits and burdens, it is permissible to forgo a life-sustaining treatment that is futile. Suppose, however, that a patient (or family member) wants, or even demands, a treatment that health care providers regard as futile. From an ethical point of view, should the treatment be provided?

The ethical principle of autonomy might be brought forward as an argument for an affirmative answer. (9, 10) According to this principle, it is the right of a patient (or his/her proxy decision maker) to make the ultimate decision about medical treatments (see chapter 1). On the other hand, it is argued that it is irresponsible and a violation of professional integrity for a health care professional to offer or provide a therapy that is unlikely to work. (11, 12) Further, such action may offer false hope to a patient (10) or even increase a patient's pain and discomfort in the final days of life. (13) On this view, patient autonomy is meaningful only when the patient is presented with a choice between medically viable options, and futile treatment is not really a viable option. (12, 14, 15) In sum:

> Although the ethical requirement to respect patient autonomy entitles a patient to choose from among medically acceptable treatment options (or to reject all options), it does not entitle patients to receive whatever treatments they ask for. Instead, the obligations of physicians are limited

to offering treatments that are consistent with professional standards of care. (13)

The last statement could be expanded beyond physicians to any health care professional.

Another dimension of the futility dilemma is determining exactly what constitutes "futile" treatment. How should medical futility be defined? The answer is surprisingly complex.

On an intuitive level, medical futility "refers to interventions that are unlikely to produce any significant benefit for the patient." (13) But how narrowly or how broadly should "benefit" for the patient be understood? In this regard, we find it useful to distinguish definitions of futility which take a *physicalist* approach from those which take a *personalist* approach.

Physicalist definitions of futility focus on the body of a patient and physiological outcomes of medical interventions. For example:

- A medical intervention is futile if the patient has a lethal diagnosis or prognosis of imminent death. (9)
- A medical intervention is futile if evidence exists that the intervention cannot achieve its physiologic goal. (9)
- A medical intervention is futile if the intervention does not work in more than one percent of attempts (16) or, otherwise stated, if it is ineffective more than 99 percent of the time. (11)
- A medical intervention is futile if evidence exists that the intervention will not or cannot extend the patient's life span. (9)

Concomitantly, a medical intervention would not be considered futile if undertaken for a patient who does not have a lethal diagnosis or who is not imminently dying. Or again, a medical intervention would not be considered futile if it can achieve its physiologic goal; for example, if resuscitation will, in fact, revive a patient. The third definition is a statistical specification of the second. (9) On the fourth definition, an intervention would not be considered futile if it had the benefit of extending a patient's life span, although what constitutes an enhanced life span is ambiguous (viz., a day, a week, a month). (9)

Personalist definitions of futility consider the broader context of a patient's life, considering not merely the patient's body but "the patient as person." (10) For example:

- A medical intervention is futile if evidence exists that the intervention will not or cannot enhance the patient's quality of life. (9)

- A medical intervention is futile if evidence exists that the intervention will not or cannot achieve the patient's or family's goals. (9)

For example, a medical intervention might prolong a patient's life (and, on a physicalist understanding of futility, not be futile treatment) but leave the patient incapable of surviving outside the intensive care unit. From a quality of life perspective, this could be considered futile treatment. (10) On the other hand, suppose that a woman who has ovarian cancer and who is close to death would like to reconcile with an estranged son before she dies. And let us suppose further that she develops pneumonia. From a physicalist perspective, using antibiotics to treat her pneumonia might be judged futile treatment on the grounds that she is imminently dying. However, if treating her with antibiotics will buy a few days time and allow her to achieve the personal goal of seeing her son, then this medical intervention would not be considered futile treatment from a personalist perspective. In sum, the various definitions of futility can yield different judgments about the futility of a medical intervention for a particular patient.

Which definition of futility should be adopted? The Council on Ethical and Judicial Affairs of the American Medical Association has taken the position that "futility is intrinsically a value judgment" and hence found "great difficulty in assigning an absolute definition to the term futile care." (16) Instead, the Council proposed a process for decision making in cases of apparent futility, a process which can be generalized beyond physicians:

- Earnest attempts should be made in advance to deliberate over and negotiate prior understandings between patient, proxy and physician on what constitutes futile care for the patient, and what falls within acceptable limits for the physician, family, and possibly also the institution.
- Joint decision-making should occur between patient or proxy and physician to the maximum extent possible.
- Attempts should be made to negotiate disagreements if they arise, and to reach resolution within all parties' acceptable limits, with the assistance of consultants as appropriate.
- Involvement of an institutional committee such as the ethics committee should be requested if disagreements are irresolvable.
- If the institutional review supports the patient's position and the physician remains unpersuaded, transfer of care to another physician within the institution may be arranged.
- If the process supports the physician's position and the patient/proxy remains unpersuaded, transfer to another institution may be sought and, if done, should be supported by the transferring and receiving institution.

- If transfer is not possible the intervention need not be offered. (16)

Noteworthy is the role assigned to an ethics committee in dealing with disputes about futility (see chapter 2). The process outlined "allows a hearing for patient and proxy assessments of worthwhile outcome" as well as for consideration of the perspectives of health care providers. (16) It is preferable to unilateral decision making on the part of a health care professional to deny a treatment which, from his or her point of view, is futile. (9) This process also has the advantage of providing a system for addressing ethical dilemmas regarding futility without the need for recourse to the court system. (16)

CHAPTER SUMMARY

Key Terms and Concepts

principle of patient autonomy: self-determination; the right of a patient to make the final decision in matters pertaining to his or her own life and health care.

principle of weighing benefits and burdens: it is morally permissible to forgo (that is, withhold or withdraw) a life-sustaining treatment if the burdens of the treatment outweigh its benefits or if the treatment is useless or futile.

Key Points

- Patients themselves, not health care providers, have the right to make the final decision about using or forgoing life-sustaining treatments. (principle of patient autonomy)
- Patients should make their decisions on the basis of considering the relative benefits and burdens of the treatment. (principle of weighing benefits and burdens)
- It is ethically permissible either to *withhold* or to *withdraw* a life-sustaining treatment.
- Withholding or withdrawing a life-sustaining treatment is *not* the same as euthanasia.
- It is ethically permissible to withhold or withdraw a treatment that is futile. Problems arise from the fact that different people understand "futility" in different ways.

FOR FURTHER DISCUSSION

1. Have you ever experienced in your family or with close friends a situation in which a decision had to be made about using or forgoing life-sustaining treatments? Describe the case and the decision that was made. Why was this particular decision made? If the decision were up to you, would you have made the same decision or a different one? Why or why not?

2. The case of Roger Smith represents a situation of family conflict regarding the use of life-sustaining treatments. Roger, the patient in question, wishes to forgo all medical treatments, and two of his children support him in making this choice. On the other hand, Roger's wife Kate and one of their daughters disagree with Roger's decision.

   In American medical ethics, a good deal of emphasis is placed on patient autonomy. Following this principle, it would be concluded that health care providers should do what Roger wants, even if family members cannot accept his decision. Some contend, however, that an exclusive emphasis on patient autonomy represents an extreme form of individualism that ignores the fact that we are involved in relationships with other people and that our actions as individuals also affect them.

   In your view, should Roger's wife and children have any say in the decision about using or forgoing medical treatments? If so, what do you think their appropriate role is? Do you think that the ethical principle of autonomy should be limited in any way?

3. The ethical theory of principalism includes the principles of autonomy, beneficence, nonmaleficence and justice (see chapter 1). Apply principalism to the treatment decisions that must be made in the case of Roger Smith. Do you reach the same or different conclusions than applying the principle of autonomy alone? Do you reach the same or different conclusions than using the principle of weighing benefits and burdens?

4. As a result of an automobile accident four months ago, Martha Miller, 54, is paralyzed from the waist down and must use a wheel chair for mobility. Since being released from the hospital, an occupational therapist, Ted Marlow, has been working with Martha to evaluate her home environment and to recommend adaptations. Martha is divorced and her two adult children live out of state, but Ted is confident that Martha will be able to live independently and even be able to continue her work as a journalist out of her home.

   However, Martha's adjustment to her new situation is complicated by the fact that she develops kidney problems. Her physician recommends starting dialysis treatment, and indicates that her prognosis is good for living at least ten more years if she begins dialysis immediately. The local Dial-a-Ride service can provide transportation for Martha to the dialysis center.

Martha tells her physician that "enough is enough" and that she just wants to be left alone.

The physician is concerned that Martha is acting out of depression, and asks for a consult with the ethics committee at the local hospital to seek guidance in handling this situation. The physician asks Ted Marlow to participate in the ethics consult as one of Martha's caregivers.

Role-play this ethics consult. Have participants assume the roles of ethics committee members, Martha's physician, Ted Marlow the occupational therapist, and Martha Miller herself.

- *Suppose that Martha is persuaded to attend the ethics consult meeting. How might she explain and justify her decision to forgo dialysis?*
- *Suppose you are Martha's physician. How might you argue in favor of Martha undertaking dialysis?*
- *Suppose that you are Ted Marlow, the occupational therapist working with Martha. As an "outsider," how do you see Martha's desire to forgo the dialysis treatment?*
- *What ethical principles should be brought forward by the members of the ethics committee to guide decision making in this case? How do these principles apply to this case? What facts about this case are important in applying these principles?*

After considering these various points of view and the ethical principles for making decisions about life-sustaining treatments, do you personally think that Martha should undertake dialysis or not? What factors in the case do you consider critical in coming to this judgment?

5. Consider the case of Elaine Manion. Dr. Lee considers resuscitation to be "futile" treatment in her case. What concept(s) of futility might underlie Dr. Lee's judgment? Could any case be made that an attempt to resuscitate Elaine should not be considered "futile" treatment? In your judgment, should an attempt to resuscitate Elaine be considered "futile" treatment?

References

1. Hastings Center, *Guidelines on the Termination of Life-Sustaining Treatment and the Care of the Dying* (Briarcliff Manor, NY: Hastings Center, 1987).
2. President's Commission for the Study of Ethical Problems in Medicine and Biomedical and Behavioral Research, *Deciding to Forego Life-Sustaining Treatment* (1983; reprint New York: Concern for Dying).
3. Benedict M. Ashley, O.P., Jean K. deBlois, C.S.J., and Kevin D. O'Rourke, O.P., *Health Care Ethics A Catholic Theological Analysis*, 5th ed. (Washington, D.C.: Georgetown University Press, 2006).
4. Joanne Lynn and James F. Childress, "Must Patients Always Be Given Food and Water?" in Joanne Lynn (ed.), *By No Extraordinary Means: The Choice to Forgo Life-Sustaining Food and Water* (Bloomington, IN: Indiana University Press, 1986).
5. Bupa, "Pneumonia," http://hcd2.bupa.co.uk/fact_sheets/html/Pneumonia.html. Accessed January 2009.
6. Palm Beach County Caring, *An Advance Directive/End of Life Plan of Care*, http://www.pbccaring.org/downloads/AdvanceDirectiveEnd%20ofLife-PlanofCareandInstructions.doc.
7. Daniel Callahan, *The Troubled Dream of Life In Search of a Peaceful Death* (New York: Simon & Schuster, 1993).
8. Mary Sawyer, "Care, Not Cure: What to Say When Treatment Fails," *Journal of Hospice and Palliative Nursing* 4/3 (July/September 2002): 133-35.
9. Committee on Ethics of the American College of Obstetricians and Gynecologists, "ACOG Committee Opinion: Medical Futility" (March 2007; reaffirmed 2008), http://www.acog.org/from_home/publications/ethics/co362.pdf. Accessed January 2009.
10. Lawrence J. Schneiderman, Nancy S. Jecker, and Albert R. Jonsen, "Medical Futility: Response to Critiques," *Annals of Internal Medicine* 125/8 (15 October 1996): 669-74.
11. Endlink Resource for End of Life Care Education, "Definitions of Medical Futility," http://endoflife/northwestern.edu/medical_futility/what.cfm#Definitions. Accessed January 2009.
12. Tom Tomlinson and Howard Brody, "Futility and the Ethics of Resuscitation," *Journal of the American Medical Association* 264/10 (September 12, 1990): 1276-80.
13. Nancy S. Jecker, "Futility," *Ethics in Medicine University of Washington School of Medicine* (1998), http://depts.washington.edu/bioethx/topics/futil.html. Accessed January 2009.

14. James Drane and John Coulehan, "The Concept of Futility: Patients Do Not Have a Right to Demand Medically Useless Treatment," *Health Progress* 74/10 (December 1993): 28-32.
15. Marcia Angell, "The Case of Helga Wanglie: A New Kind of 'Right to Die' Case," *New England Journal of Medicine* 325 (1991): 511-12.
16. Council on Ethical and Judicial Affairs of the American Medical Association, "Medical Futility in End-of-Life Care" (1996), http://www.ama-assn.org/ama1/pub/upload/mm/369/ceja_2i96.pdf. Accessed January 2009.

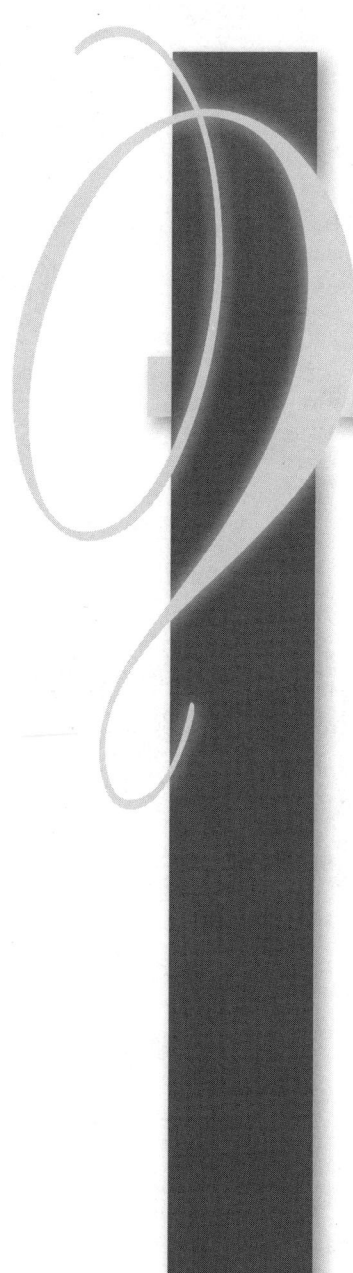

Chapter 7

Proxy Decision Making and Advance Directives

Patient Roger Smith (chapter 6) is still able to make his own health care decisions. But suppose that, in addition to cancer and pneumonia, Roger was also suffering from dementia. Who should make the decisions about continuing or discontinuing chemotherapy and about providing or refusing the doctor's recommended treatments for pneumonia? And on what basis should these decisions be made?

These questions lead to consideration of advance directives. An *advance directive* is a legal document in which an individual makes provision for future medical treatment decisions in the event that he or she loses decision-making capacity. There are two basic types of advance directive: the *living will* and the *durable power of attorney for health care*. These documents may be called by various names in different states.

Chapter Seven

In this chapter you will learn:

- who can serve as a proxy decision maker;
- how a proxy should make treatment decisions;
- what a living will says and when it goes into effect;
- what a durable power of attorney for health care does and how it differs from a living will;
- how to execute advance directives;
- what requirements for advance directives are set by federal law;
- the advantages of having advance directives;
- problems with advance directives;
- types of advance care planning other than traditional advance directives.

Case Study

Mel Langley taught math for twenty years at Elkader Community College before taking early retirement two years ago. Since his retirement, Mel has remained so active that his friends from the college joke that he has "flunked retirement." Mel is an avid reader, checking out a new set of books from the library every week. He has resumed playing the piano, something he had to give up because of the time demands of his job. He is a regular volunteer at the local senior center, and continues to tutor students in math at the college. During the summer, he travels around the country attending Elderhostel programs.

Recently, Jim Parker, Mel's friend who also taught math at the college, was diagnosed with cancer. Over a period of a year, Mel visits Jim twice a week. Mel watches Jim suffer from chemotherapy treatments and undergo repeated hospitalization. His weight loss is significant. At Jim's funeral, Mel comments that Jim doesn't even "look like himself" any more.

Jim's death causes Mel to wonder what would happen if he should be diagnosed with a terminal illness. In order to protect himself against lingering in a debilitated condition, Mel decides to make out advance directives—both a living will and a durable power of attorney for health care document. Mel never married, but he has two sisters and a younger brother. Mel names his brother as his proxy decision maker in executing his advance directives.

One Sunday morning while attending church services, Mel begins to experience severe chest pains. He is taken to the emergency room of the local hospital, where he is diagnosed as having suffered a fairly severe heart attack.

During his stay in the cardiac care unit of the hospital, Mel is given a thorough physical. It is discovered that he has prostate cancer. Mel's physician, Dr. Reynolds, thinks the condition is curable with radiation therapy. He contacts Barbara O'Connor, a radiation therapist at the hospital, to inquire when Mel could be fit into the hospital's radiation therapy program.

Medications being administered to Mel for his heart condition have left him confused, and Dr. Reynolds does not think that he has the capacity at this point to make sound decisions about his health care. For this reason, Dr. Reynolds contacts Mel's brother to authorize the treatment for prostate cancer. Dr. Reynolds wants to begin the treatment regimen as soon as Mel is stronger.

To Dr. Reynolds surprise, his brother produces Mel's advance directives and says that nothing should be done for Mel's prostate cancer. He even raises the possibility of having Mel discharged from the cardiac care unit and taken home to die. "Mel would never want to live like this," his brother states, "where he can no longer do what he used to enjoy."

Dr. Reynolds does not agree with Mel's brother. He does not think that Mel is "at the brink of death." To be sure, Mel's heart problems will leave him with a more restricted life style, but that is not the same as being terminally ill. And his prostate cancer is very likely curable.

Mel's two sisters also come to see him, and approach Dr. Reynolds about his prognosis. They too disagree with the judgment of Mel's brother. At this point, they feel everything possible should be done to save Mel's life.

Dr. Reynolds decides to arrange a meeting with Mel's brother and two sisters to try to resolve the dispute. He invites Barbara O'Connor to attend in order to help explain the projected radiation therapy to Mel's family.

Barbara has recently completed her training in radiation therapy and is a new employee at the hospital. She has heard about the conflicts that can occur between physicians and family members over treatment decisions, and among members of the same family. This is the first time she has personally witnessed a conflict where a patient's very life is at stake. She wonders who is right, and how the advance directives will play out in this situation.

■ ■ ■

Proxy Decision Making

First of all, the case of Mel Langley represents a situation in which someone other than the patient must be called upon to make the medical treatment decisions because the patient himself is presently suffering from confusion due to his medications. Someone who makes health care decisions for a patient who is not mentally competent to do so is referred to as a *proxy (or surrogate) decision maker.*

This role is often assumed by the patient's next of kin, but another relative, or a close friend, or an individual who knows the patient well may serve in this capacity. Often one of these individuals naturally emerges as the proxy decision maker. For example, if Mel were married, it would be natural for his wife to be called upon to make treatment decisions on his behalf. However, it is also possible for a patient to go beyond these informal arrangements and to select in advance an individual who will be legally recognized as his proxy decision maker. This is done by executing the legal document known as a *durable power of attorney for health care* (or as a *medical power of attorney*). In our case scenario, Mel Langley executed this document and legally named his younger brother as his proxy decision maker. If a patient has not executed this document, it is possible for a court to appoint a guardian to serve legally as the patient's proxy decision maker.

From an ethical point of view, how should a proxy decision maker go about making his decision on behalf of the patient? The preferred standard for proxy decision making is *substituted judgment*. According to this standard, the proxy decision maker attempts to reach the decision that the incapacitated person would make if he or she were able to choose. (1) Thus the proxy decision maker is guided by any explicit directives given by the patient, in writing or orally in conversation. (2) If the patient has not left any explicit directives about the treatment in question, the proxy applies what is known about the patient's beliefs, values, preferences, and life-long behavior patterns to try to determine what the patient would have wanted. (2)

There are some cases in which the principle of substituted judgment cannot be applied. This is so if the patient has never been mentally competent during his lifetime and thus was never able to express any preferences. This is also the case if the patient never in fact expressed any views about the treatment in question and no longer has any close living relatives or friends who know him well enough to make predictions about his wishes. In such cases, the *best interests standard* may be used. According to this standard, the proxy decision maker tries "to make a choice for the patient that seeks to implement what is in that person's best interests by reference to more objective, societally shared criteria." (1) This standard "does not rest on the value of self-determination but solely on protection of patients' welfare." (1) It is sometimes expressed as choosing as a reasonable person in the patient's circumstances would. (2)

It is important to keep in mind that substituted judgment is the preferred standard for proxy decision making whenever it can be used. Making decisions in accord with the wishes and values of the patient represents an extension of patient autonomy to cases in which a patient cannot directly say what she wants.

The Living Will

In applying the standard of substituted judgment, a proxy decision maker should look first to any instructions the patient has made explicit in writing through the execution of advance directives.

The first type of advance directive that was developed is the living will. A living will typically goes into effect when the patient is suffering from an *incurable or irreversible disease* and is *expected to die within a short period of time*. In some states, the condition of permanent unconsciousness is also included in the scope of the living will. A living will basically says that the patient does not want life-sustaining treatments used in these circumstances. In such cases, life-sustaining treatments would not help improve the condition of the patient, but would only prolong the dying process. However, comfort care and pain medication will still be provided to the patient.

Some people are afraid to sign a living will because they think they will automatically be denied treatment in the case of any medical emergency. This is not true. For example, if someone with a living will is in a car accident and is taken to the hospital emergency room and can recover, this document will not prevent her from receiving treatment to aid in the recovery.

It is important to keep in mind that a living will goes into effect only when an individual no longer has the capacity to make his own decisions. If someone is in the final stages of the dying process but is conscious and lucid, he should still be asked directly what he does and does not want done in terms of medical treatments.

Durable Power of Attorney for Health Care

Because of limitations in the living will, another form of advance directive was developed; namely, the durable power of attorney for health care.

The language of a living will document usually gives only general directives about life-sustaining treatments. When signing such a document, an individual cannot foresee all the particular conditions which will prevail when the use of life-sustaining treatments becomes an issue in his own case. In order to provide for better decision making, a durable power of attorney for health care allows an individual to designate legally someone to make treatment decisions on his behalf when he is no longer able to do so. The legally designated proxy can engage in give-and-take discussion of medical alternatives. It is also possible to designate someone as an alternate proxy decision maker should the designated proxy be unavailable at the time a treatment decision must be made.

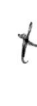

The durable power of attorney for health care is broader in scope than a living will. It goes into effect in any situation in which the patient becomes incapable of making treatment decisions, even temporarily. It is not limited to cases in which death is imminent. Suppose that an individual—let's call him Jerome—has executed this document naming his wife Beth as his legal proxy. And suppose that Jerome gets into a car accident, suffers a concussion and broken ribs, and is taken to the hospital unconscious. Beth will have the legal authority to make any needed treatment decisions on Jerome's behalf. And when Jerome regains consciousness and decision-making capacity, the right to make treatment decisions will go back to him.

The person designated as the proxy decision maker through a durable power of attorney for health care *legally* has the right to make treatment decisions and even takes precedence over (other) relatives of the patient. Many families are not aware of this. The designated proxy may (and probably should) consult with the patient's (other) relatives to try to achieve agreement on the course of action to be taken. However, the designated proxy legally has the final say about what happens.

A durable power of attorney for health care document may include a space in which the person executing the document may write in instructions about specific treatments that he does or does not want in a particular circumstance; for example, instructions about resuscitation, dialysis, chemotherapy, antibiotics, or assisted nutrition and hydration. The designated proxy is expected to act in accord with such instructions.

It is also important to keep in mind that a durable power of attorney for health care is a different legal document than a power of attorney for financial matters. The individual designated to take care of someone else's finances does *not* automatically have the power to make medical decisions for that individual.

Executing Advance Directives

A living will or a durable power of attorney for health care can only be executed by someone who is mentally competent and of legal age to do so. An adult suffering from dementia who has not already executed an advance directive can no longer do so. Similarly, adults who have suffered from severe mental deficiencies since birth cannot execute advance directives.

A person can only execute an advance directive for himself or herself. So, for example, a wife cannot executive an advance directive for a husband suffering from dementia. A parent cannot execute an advance directive for a son or daughter, even for an adult child who is incapacitated and being cared for by the parents. In such cases, a court may be asked to officially appoint a relative (or another person) as *guardian* of the patient to make treatment decisions for the patient, or often family members close to the patient simply make such decisions.

It is not absolutely necessary to see a lawyer to execute a living will or durable power of attorney for health care. Health care facilities have individuals on staff trained to provide assistance in making out these documents, usually in social services or pastoral care.

At the present time, there is no federal legislation establishing the living will and durable power of attorney for health care for the entire United States, or establishing a standard form for executing them. Legally, these documents have been established state by state. Basically, the content of them is the same, but there may be differences among various states on such matters as who may witness the document, notarization rather than witnessing, or restrictions on who may be named as the proxy decision maker. In some states, individuals may be required to give explicit directions about assisted nutrition and hydration or about treatment in a condition of permanent unconsciousness.

Thus the question arises of whether an advance directive written in one state will be recognized in other states. The Commission on Legal Problems of the Elderly of the American Bar Association has given this response:

> Many states expressly recognize out-of-state advance directives if the directive meets either the legal requirements of the state where executed or the state where the treatment decision arises. Several states are silent on this question. If there is doubt, the rules of the state where treatment takes place, not the state where the advance directive was signed, will normally control. (3)

The Commission advises that "even if an advance directive fails to meet technicalities of state law, health providers still should value the directive as important, if not controlling, evidence of the patient's wishes." (3)

While the original of an advance directive should be kept in a safe place, advance directives are not meant to be hidden. Copies of advance directives should be given to the patient's physician, family members, and proxy decision maker. The provisions of these documents should be discussed with them so that they feel comfortable with the instructions about treatment. It is also good to give a copy of advance directives to the hospital the person uses to have on record in the event of admission. Copies should also be provided to other health care facilities and services the patient is using (for example, a nursing home or hospice program). It may also be a good idea to give copies to close friends and neighbors, since these are sometimes the first individuals to find someone at home undergoing a health care crisis. Some people also keep a reduced size photocopy of their advance directives in their wallets.

Advance directives are not just for senior citizens. They are useful for any adult to have. In fact, several well-known court cases about the withdrawal of life-sustaining treatments—the cases of Karen Ann Quinlan, Nancy Cruzan, and Terri Schiavo—involved young adults in their twenties and thirties! (4)

Advance directive documents can be changed or even revoked. They should be reviewed periodically to ensure that they still reflect the wishes of the person who has executed them.

The Patient Self-Determination Act

Federal legislation, called the *Patient Self-Determination Act,* has established requirements regarding advance directives for health care providers receiving Medicare and/or Medicaid funding. Specifically, the legislation sets the following requirements:

- A health care facility or agency must provide written information to each adult concerning his or her rights under state law to make decisions concerning medical care. This should include information about the right to accept or refuse medical or surgical treatment and the right to formulate advance directives.
- A health care facility or service must have written policies respecting the implementation of these rights.
- A health care facility or service must inquire in the case of each adult whether she has an advance directive.
- Documentation must be made in the patient's medical record whether he has executed an advance directive.
- A health care facility or service cannot condition the provision of care or otherwise discriminate against an individual based on whether she has executed an advance directive.
- A health care facility or service must comply with the requirements of state laws respecting advance directives.

- Health care facilities and services must provide education on advance directives for staff and for the community at large. (5)

The law does *not* require a health care facility or agency to carry out any directive whatever contained in a living will or durable power of attorney for health care. No facility or agency is required to act contrary to its mission and ethical values, even if a patient requests this in writing. However, a facility or service must provide written policies specifying the limits on the procedures it will perform. And a clear summary of the facility's or service's policies regarding advance directives and consent to or refusal of medical treatment must be available to the public. (5)

It is very important to recognize that the Patient Self-Determination Act does *not* require anyone to execute advance directives, but only requires that patients be informed that these documents are available for their use.

Finally, health care workers may be required to attend in-service programs on advance directives. Such educational programs for the staff of a health care facility or service are mandated by the Patient Self-Determination Act. (5)

Advantages of Advance Directives

Autonomy (self-determination) is a value much emphasized in health care today. Advance directives are a way of extending the ethical value of patient autonomy. They allow a patient to control medical treatment decision making when she no longer has the ability to state her wishes directly. Advance directives are also regarded as a way of preventing the overuse of life-sustaining treatments. People have seen the lives of family members and friends prolonged in a much debilitated state, and their response is, "I would never want that to happen to me!" Indeed, in the case scenario of Mel Langley, it is Mel's experience of a friend dying of cancer that prompts him to execute advance directives.

We live in a litigious society. Health care providers may sometimes be reluctant to withhold or withdraw life-sustaining treatments for fear of being legally liable. However, if an advance directive has been executed and the health care provider acts in accord with it in not providing life-sustaining treatments, the health care provider has protection. (6) Thus, advance directives can make health care providers more comfortable about complying with requests to forgo life-sustaining treatments.

Advance directives can also be useful when conflicts arise among family members or between family members and health care providers. In such circumstances, if a durable power of attorney for health care has been executed, the designated proxy legally has the power to make the final decision and bring the conflict to resolution. Executing advance directives can prevent conflicts from going to court for resolution.

Problems with Advance Directives

Through a living will, an individual indicates a desire to forgo life-sustaining treatments when death is near. An individual may also give directions about types of treatments that are or are not wanted in a variety of circumstances in a durable power of attorney for health care document. But can anyone accurately predict how she will *feel* in such circumstances? For example, when a person is healthy and active, she may view life with a serious, debilitating illness as unacceptable. But when she is actually in such a condition, holding on to life may appear very different. (For example, what is your own reaction to the possibility of suffering an accident that would leave you a quadriplegic in a wheelchair? And might you change your mind if this actually happened to you?)

Another problem concerns how to write instructions included in advance directives. Let's suppose that someone—let's call him Ben—has prepared advance directives stipulating that "under no circumstances" does he want to be hooked up to a breathing machine "for any illness." And let's further suppose that Ben subsequently suffers from delirium and Guillain-Barré syndrome (a potentially reversible illness causing progressive weakness and paralysis) and that Ben's physician recommends to his wife, Thelma, that he be placed on a ventilator, telling her that there is a 60 percent chance of full recovery with temporary mechanical support. Thelma knows the instructions Ben gave in his advance directives. She also believes that, when Ben gave these instructions, he thought that being connected to a ventilator meant that he would merely have biological functioning sustained indefinitely with no chance of recovery. She thinks that if Ben knew he had a chance of recovery by being placed on a ventilator, he would take it. (5)

This case illustrates the point that, in making out an advance directive, an individual cannot envision all of the possible types of circumstances he might be in. Thus in writing an advance directive, one should not make instructions so specific or absolute as to preclude administration of medically beneficial treatment.

A complication in writing instructions for forgoing life-sustaining treatments is a legal trend to want "clear and convincing evidence" that a patient would not want the treatment in the particular situation in which he is found. (7, 8) Again, an individual cannot envision all of the various circumstances he might be in medically when making out an advance directive, much less give detailed instructions for the various scenarios. A possible way of circumventing this problem is to include a statement in a durable power of attorney for health care document to the effect that, if one's wishes are not clear about using or forgoing a particular treatment in a particular circumstance, one wants one's designated proxy to use his or her judgment about what would be in one's best interests.

There are several problems health care providers may encounter in using advance directives. For one thing, patients may say they have these documents but forget to bring them to the health care facility or service so that they can be placed in the medical record and actually guide treatment decision-making. Or again, it may not be understood that an advance directive is *not* the same thing as a Do-Not-Resuscitate Order, which must be written by a physician. Another common problem is that family members do not understand the legal status of the proxy decision maker named through a durable power of attorney for health care; namely, that this individual has the final decision regarding medical treatment and takes precedence over any (other) relative. This lack of understanding can result in family conflict. Or again, it may be unclear whether an individual still has the mental competency to make medical treatment decisions and, concomitantly, it will be unclear whether an advance directive should become operative.

The durable power of attorney for health care carries its own special problems. It is not unusual for an individual to ask a family member to serve as his proxy decision maker. However, it may be emotionally difficult for this family member to make a decision to "let go" of a loved one by forgoing life-sustaining treatments, even though this is what the individual in question would have wanted. In other words, acting as a proxy decision maker for medical treatments can prove a burdensome task to assume. (6)

Further, residents of advanced age in long-term care facilities may have outlived the family members and friends who would be candidates for selection as their proxy decision maker. And if they have no one to designate to serve in this capacity, they are precluded from executing this type of advance directive. (6)

Other Types of Advance Care Planning

Documents for advance care planning are not limited to those enacted by state legislation. One such document is the *Five Wishes*. (9) This document includes not only the medical wishes but also the personal, emotional and spiritual wishes of seriously ill persons. (10) Its five sections cover "The Person I Want to Make Care Decisions for Me When I Can't," "The Kind of Medical Treatment I Want or Don't Want," "How Comfortable I Want to Be," "How I Want People to Treat

Me," and "What I Want My Loved Ones to Know." Like the durable power of attorney for health care document, it allows one to designate a proxy decision maker. Like the living will, it allows one to give instructions regarding medical treatments at the very end of life. However, it goes beyond these two documents in offering choices about non-medical means of comfort care (e.g., being massaged with warm oils, having favorite music played, having religious readings and poems read aloud), about the environment in which one is to die (e.g., dying at home, having pictures of loved ones in one's room, having one's hand held and being talked to by others, having others by one's side praying), and about one's final communications to others (e.g., that one loves and forgives other people, how one wants to be remembered, one's desires for funeral services). The *Five Wishes* document is recognized as a legally valid advance directive in most states. (11)

The POLST (Physician Orders for Life-Sustaining Treatment) Paradigm Initiative is coordinated by the Center for Ethics in Health Care at Oregon Health and Sciences University. (12) This project has provided a model form which is being used in various states, with some modifications and refinements of the template. (13) The POLST form and its variants translate a patient's values and wishes, whether expressed personally, by a proxy decision maker, or in an advance directive, into *actual physician orders*. (14, 15, 16) This directive for patient care is portable across health care services—hospital, long-term care, home care, hospice, EMT services. (14, 15, 16, 17, 18) Sections of the form address resuscitation, the use of antibiotics, the use of assisted nutrition and hydration, and choices regarding comfort measures only versus various levels of medical interventions, including transfer to a hospital or intensive care unit. (13, 14, 18, 19) The POLST form is intended for seriously ill persons with life-limiting illnesses, for those who are chronically ill, and for residents of long-term care facilities (15, 16, 17), and is meant to be reviewed periodically to reflect the current condition of the patient. (13) As an instrument for advance care planning, POLST is very promising. It has been noted that "a decade of research in Oregon has proven that the POLST Program more accurately conveys end-of-life preferences and yields higher adherence by medical professionals." (17) Or again, "key findings indicate that the patients' values are accurately reflected by the orders, that the orders are followed by first responders, that life-sustaining treatment orders beyond CPR (e.g., artificial nutrition) are useful, and that implementation can evolve to become a standard of care." (14)

CHAPTER SUMMARY

Key Terms and Concepts

principle of substituted judgment: a proxy decision maker attempts to reach the decision that the incapacitated person would make if he or she were able to choose, relying on written or oral directives explicitly given by the patient or on knowledge of the patient's beliefs, values, preferences, and life-long behavior patterns.

best interests standard: a proxy decision maker makes a choice that seeks to implement what is in the patient's best interests by reference to objective, societally shared criteria. It is sometimes expressed as choosing as a reasonable person in the patient's circumstances would.

advance directive: a legal document in which an individual makes provision for future medical treatment decisions in the event that he or she loses decision-making capacity.

living will: one type of advance directive in which an individual gives instructions to forgo life-sustaining treatments when he or she is suffering from an incurable or irreversible illness and death is imminent (and, in some states, when he or she is in a state of permanent unconsciousness).

durable power of attorney for health care: one type of advance directive in which an individual legally designates someone as his or her proxy decision maker for times when he or she is incapacitated and cannot make treatment decisions.

Key Points

- When a patient is no longer capable of making treatment decisions, a proxy decision maker acts on behalf of the patient. An individual may be legally designated as the proxy decision maker through a durable power of attorney for health care document, or as a court appointed guardian.
- Whenever possible, a proxy decision maker should make treatment decisions on the basis of what the patient himself or herself would want done *(principle of substituted judgment)*.
- There are two types of legally recognized advance directives: the *living will* and the *durable power of attorney for health care*. These documents can be executed by mentally competent persons of legal age, but only for themselves.
- The living will is *not* applicable to medical emergencies from which a patient can recover with appropriate treatment. It goes into effect only when the

patient is suffering from an incurable or irreversible illness, and death is imminent, and the patient has lost the capacity to make his or her own treatment decisions. In some states, a living will also applies to patients who are permanently unconscious.

- A durable power of attorney for health care provides for a proxy decision maker who can assess the specific condition of the patient and engage in give-and-take discussion of medical alternatives. It is broader in scope than a living will, going into effect whenever a patient becomes incapacitated to make his or her own decisions, even temporarily.
- At the present time the living will and durable power of attorney for health care documents are legally established by individual states. Generally, one can expect an advance directive executed in one state to be honored in other states.
- The federal Patient Self-Determination Act requires all health care facilities and agencies to provide information about advance directives to patients, to inquire whether he or she has executed one, and to record the response on the patient's medical record. The law does *not* require anyone to execute an advance directive, but does require that health care facilities and agencies let people know that these documents are available if they wish to use them.
- Advance directives are beneficial in promoting patient autonomy, protecting against the overuse of life-sustaining treatments, making health care providers more comfortable with complying with requests to forgo life-sustaining treatments, and helping to resolve conflicts about using or forgoing treatments without going to court.
- Challenges in using advance directives include projecting what one would and would not want done in types of health situations one may never have experienced, and the fact that one cannot envision all the possible scenarios in which medical treatment decisions may have to be made. In giving treatment instructions, some room should be left for discretionary judgment.
- There are documents for advance care planning in addition to those established by state legislation, such as the *Five Wishes* document and *POLST* (Physician's Order for Life-Sustaining Treatment).

FOR FURTHER DISCUSSION

1. Consider the case of Mel Langley at the beginning of the chapter. The physician Dr. Reynolds arranges a meeting to discuss the course of action to be taken.

Role play this meeting. Participants should assume the roles of Dr. Reynolds, Mel's brother, Mel's two sisters, and radiation therapist Barbara O'Connor. The following points should be included in the conversation.

- Mel has executed a living will. Does it go into effect in his present condition?
- Mel has executed a durable power of attorney for health care. Does it go into effect in his present condition?
- Who should make the decision about using/forgoing medical treatments for Mel?
- What principles should be used in arriving at a decision about using/forgoing medical treatments for Mel? And how do they apply to Mel's case?
- Is there any other factual information that is needed to make a good decision?

After listening to this conversation, what do you think should be done about using/forgoing medical treatments for Mel?

2. Obtain copies of the living will and durable power of attorney for health care for your state. In small groups, review these documents. Do you have any questions about the content of these documents? About how to fill them out?
3. Do you know you anyone who has executed an advance directive? How did the person feel about doing this? Do you know of any cases in which an advance directive was used in making treatment decisions?

References

1. President's Commission for the Study of Ethical Problems in Medicine and Biomedical and Behavioral Research, *Deciding to Forego Life-Sustaining Treatment* (1983; reprint New York: Concern for Dying).
2. Hastings Center, *Guidelines on the Termination of Life-Sustaining Treatment and the Care of the Dying* (Briarcliff Manor, NY: Hastings Center, 1987).
3. Commission on Legal Problems of the Elderly of the American Bar Association, "10 Legal Myths about Advance Directives," http://www.aba-net.org/elderly/myths.html. Accessed January 2009.
4. Gregory E. Pence, *Medical Ethics Accounts of the Cases That Shaped and Define Medical Ethics*, 5th ed. (New York: McGraw-Hill, 2008).

5. Catholic Health Association of the United States, *The Patient Self-Determination Act* (St. Louis: Catholic Health Association, 1991).
6. Nancy M.P. King, *Making Sense of Advance Directives,* rev. ed. (Washington, DC: Georgetown University Press, 1996).
7. George J. Annas, "'Culture of Life' Politics at the Bedside The Case of Terri Schiavo," in Arthur Caplan, James J. McCartney, and Dominic A. Sisti (eds.), *The Case of Terri Schiavo* (Amherst, NY: Prometheus Books, 2006).
8. Timothy E. Quill, "Terri Schiavo—A Tragedy Compounded," in Arthur Caplan, James J. McCartney, and Dominic A. Sisti (eds.), *The Case of Terri Schiavo* (Amherst, NY: Prometheus Books, 2006).
9. Aging with Dignity. P.O. Box 1661, Tallahassee, Florida 32302-1661; tel. 888-594-7437; http://www.fivewishes@agingwithdignity.org.
10. Aging with Dignity, *Five Wishes,* http://www.agingwithdignity.org/5wishes.html. Accessed January 2009.
11. Learning Place Online, *Five Wishes,* http://www.learningplaceonline.com/stages/together/wishes/wishes-1.htm. Accessed January 2009.
12. Center for Ethics in Health Care, Oregon Health and Sciences University, *POLST,* http://www.ohsu.edu/ethics/polst. Accessed January 2009.
13. Center for Ethics in Health Care, Oregon Health and Sciences University, *POLST,* http://www.ohsu.edu/ethics/polst/programs/sample-forms.htm. Accessed January 2009.
14. Patrick Dunn, Alvin H. Moss, and Susan Tolle, *Fast Fact and Concept #178 The National POLST Paradigm,* http://www.eperc.mcw.edu/fastFact/ff_178.htm. Accessed January 2009.
15. Patricia A. Bomba, *Medical Orders for Life-Sustaining Treatments MOLST Staff Education,* http://www.ohsu.edu/ethics/polst/resources/docs/molst.ppt. Accessed January 2009.
16. Patricia Bomba, *Advance Care Planning: Where Does MOLST fit?* http://www.ohsu.edu/ethics/polst/resources/docs/molst+fit.pdf. Accessed January 2009.
17. Patricia Bomba, *Honoring Preferences, The Role of MOLST Medical Orders for Life-Sustaining Treatment,* http://www.ohsu.edu/ethics/polst/resources/docs/molst+open.pdf. Accessed January 2009.
18. Terri Schmidt, *POLST: Respecting Patient Wishes near the End of Life.* http://www.ohsu.edu/ethics/polst/developing/docs/polst+and+ems+rev3.ppt. Accessed January 2009.
19. Colorado Advance Directives Consortium, *Portability of Advance Directives and the Colorado Medical Orders for Scope of Treatment,* http://www.state.co.us/gov_dir/leg_dir/lcsstaff/2008/comsched/08HCTF0905AttachA.pdf. Accessed January 2009.

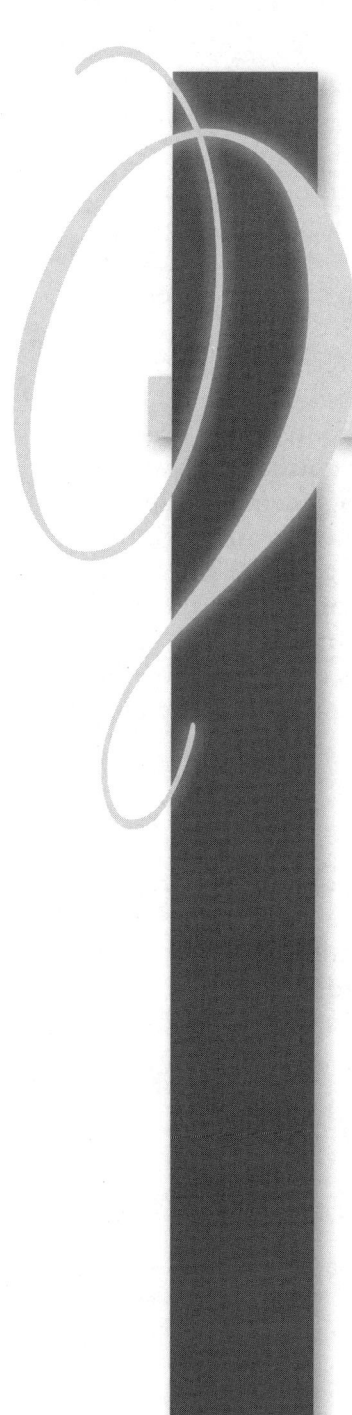

Chapter 8

The Dilemma of Assisted Nutrition and Hydration

After an automobile accident at age 24, Nancy Cruzan entered a vegetative state. She was permanently unconscious, unaware of her surroundings, unable to communicate, and unable to chew or swallow in a normal manner. After four years in this condition in a Missouri hospital, Nancy's family requested that the feeding tube that was keeping her alive be removed and that she be allowed to die. A court order, granting permission to withdraw the feeding tube, was overturned on appeal to the Missouri State Supreme Court. The question of removing Nancy's feeding tube eventually went to the United States Supreme Court. (1) Both legally and ethically, the issue of withholding or withdrawing tube feeding has been so controversial that it deserves special attention among life-sustaining treatments.

What is known as *artificial nutrition and hydration* or (*medically*) *assisted nutrition and hydration* can take various forms. A needle may be inserted into a vein in the arm; this is known as *peripheral intravenous feeding*. Or a catheter may be inserted into a central vein near the heart, which is called *central intravenous feeding* or *total parenteral feeding* or *hyperalimentation.* Another form is the *nasogastric (NG) tube,* which consists of a thin plastic tube inserted through the nose into the stomach or into the first portion of the duodenum. A *gastrostomy tube* is inserted directly into the stomach, either surgically or through an incision made with the assistance of an endoscope (PEG—percutaneous endoscopic gastrostomy). A *jejunostomy tube* is placed in the small intestine, either surgically or by a method similar to PEG tube placement. (2, 3)

Assisted nutrition and hydration may be used on a short-term basis following surgery when the patient temporarily cannot eat. (2) Such uses of assisted nutrition and hydration are not controversial. But assisted nutrition and hydration can also be used for longer periods of time in a variety of circumstances in which the patient cannot get adequate nutrition and hydration by normal means. A patient may be unable to swallow because of a stroke. Cancers can block the gastrointestinal tract. Enzymes necessary to absorb nutrients in the intestines may be inadequate. Or, while the patient may have a normal mouth, stomach, and intestinal tract, she may be adverse to or uninterested in eating. (2) From an ethical point of view, assisted nutrition and hydration has been controversial when used for a prolonged period of time as a means (and sometimes the only means) of continuing to keep a patient alive.

In this chapter you will learn about:

- the controversy surrounding whether assisted nutrition and hydration should be classified as "standard care" or as "medical treatment";
- the benefits and burdens of assisted nutrition and hydration;
- common misunderstandings about assisted nutrition and hydration;
- guidelines developed by the American Dietetic Association for providing assisted nutrition and hydration.

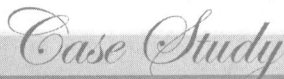

> Barbara Ryan, a 70 year-old-widow, is the kind of grandmother whose life revolves around her grandchildren. She is constantly doing things with them and taking them places. Barbara has always enjoyed reasonably good health. Everyone is surprised when she collapses at a church picnic to which she has taken three of her grandchildren.

At the hospital, Barbara's daughter Ann and son Robert are told that Barbara has suffered a stroke. Because of this, she cannot swallow normally. Ann and Robert have no qualms about consenting to the placement of the feeding tube for their mother.

After a week, Barbara is transferred to the Forest Glen Nursing Home. Her family visits her frequently. Because Barbara's grandchildren are anxious for her to get well, Barbara's daughter and son insist that her physician and the nursing home staff do everything necessary for her recovery.

However, Barbara eventually lapses into a semiconscious state. She doesn't recognize family members or friends when they come to visit her. She is bedridden, listless, and suffers periodic bouts of aspiration pneumonia caused by the feeding tube.

After their mother has been in this condition for two years, Ann and Robert begin to reassess their directive to the physician and nursing home staff to "do everything" for their mother. They recall a statement she made while taking care of their dying father. She said most emphatically that she was "ready to die when God wanted to take her" and wanted "no heroic measures to interfere with God's plan."

Ann goes to court to be named her mother's legal guardian. With the agreement of her brother, Ann requests that the tube feeding that is keeping their mother alive be stopped. Barbara's physician agrees to this request.

However, the facility's dietitian, Ron Kennedy, who has been involved in Barbara's care for the past two years, becomes very upset when he hears that Barbara's feeding tube will be removed. He believes it is wrong to deny any person food and water. In fact, Ron tells the facility's administrator that, if Barbara's feeding tube is removed, he will have to consider quitting his job because he does not want to be part of a resident being "starved to death."

■ ■ ■

"Standard Care" or "Medical Treatment"?

The dietitian in our case believes that it is wrong to deny any person food and water. One issue that arose early in the debate about assisted nutrition and hydration is whether it should be classified as "standard nursing care" and hence should always be provided, or whether it should be regarded as a "medical treatment" to be used or forgone on the same basis as other life-sustaining treatments.

Those who regard assisted nutrition and hydration as standard nursing care have put forward several arguments in support of their view. They point out that, while medical treatment is therapeutic, nutrition and hydration are not because they will not cure a disease. (4, 5) However, it could be said in rebuttal that not all recognized medical treatments cure disease. For example, kidney dialysis does not cure the problem of kidney failure, but simply provides a way of circumventing the problem. Similarly, assisted nutrition and hydration circumvents problems with eating.

It has also been argued that withholding or withdrawing food and fluids is different than withholding or withdrawing medical therapies because of its finality. Withholding or withdrawing food and fluids ensures death, whereas in the case of removing a patient from a ventilator, for example, the patient may surprise us and breathe on her own. (4, 5, 6, 7) However, this line of argument ignores the fact that stopping dialysis inevitably results in a patient's death, as does a decision not to perform cardiopulmonary resuscitation when a cardiac arrest occurs. (8) Moreover, in the case of an unconscious patient, a ventilator and assisted nutrition and hydration are alike in that both replace normal bodily functions that are compromised by that patient's illness. (9)

Some assisted feeding devices are surgically inserted, and this is certainly a medical procedure. In addition, assisted nutrition and hydration is used by a physician's order, and is monitored by a physician or someone working under a physician's direction. (9)

In the case of Nancy Cruzan, the U.S. Supreme Court took the position that her feeding tube was a "medical procedure." (10) Similarly, the American Dietetic Association has taken the position that assisted nutrition and hydration is to be considered a "medical intervention." (11) On this view, using or forgoing assisted nutrition and hydration is decided on the same basis as using or forgoing other medical life-sustaining procedures, viz., considering the benefits and burdens of the procedure and the wishes of the patient (see chapter 6).

In 2004 the question of the status of assisted nutrition and hydration was resurrected by an address given by Pope John Paul II to a conference on vegetative state patients (see chapter 9) held at the Vatican. John Paul II stated the view that "the administration of water and food, even when provided by artificial means, always represents a natural means of preserving life, not a medical act." (12) A subsequent clarification of this papal address from the Vatican Congregation for the Doctrine of the Faith reaffirmed this view but indicated that assisted nutrition and hydration may be forgone for a patient in a vegetative state if this procedure is not effective in providing the patient with nourishment or if the procedure proves excessively burdensome for the patient. (13) This is not a contradictory position because, within Catholic moral theology, early discussions of "extraordinary," non-obligatory treatments "did not necessarily concern medical acts per se, but also included actions like moving one's residence to a more suitable climate and the use of 'delicate' foods." (14; see also 15)

Yet another position on the status of assisted nutrition and hydration is that it is a combination of both medical treatment and basic health care: the method by which nutrition and hydration is delivered is a medical procedure but the material conveyed (food and water) belongs to the category of basic health care. (15) Otherwise stated:

> In itself, the provision of food and water (by whatever means) is the ordinary way of sustaining a patient's life and a minimal part of the care we owe to others. . . . While the act of feeding a person is not itself a medical act, the insertion of a tube, monitoring of the tube and patient, and prescription of the substances to be provided, do involve a degree of medical and/or nursing expertise. To insert a feeding tube is a medical decision subject to the normal criteria for medical intervention. (16)

This position likewise admits the permissibility of forgoing assisted nutrition and hydration if it proves futile or excessively burdensome. (15, 16)

A common denominator in the categorization of assisted nutrition and hydration as a medical treatment, in the position of the Vatican, and in the position that assisted nutrition and hydration is a combination of medical treatment and basic health care, is a recognition that it is legitimate to forgo this procedure in some cases and that this may be determined using the principle of weighing benefits and burdens.

The Benefits and Burdens of Assisted Nutrition and Hydration

Assisted nutrition and hydration can have distinct benefits for some patients. It offers the very fundamental benefit of "prolonging life in patients who are unable to take adequate nutrition by mouth." (17) It can also benefit patients by providing time to treat underlying medical problems or to clarify the patient's prognosis. (17) Assisted nutrition and hydration may help to stabilize a patient's physical status following severe trauma. (18) It may allow a restful healing time for a diseased or damaged gastrointestinal tract, or serve as a means to provide nutrition and hydration during a restoration period following surgery. (18) It can serve to reverse malnutrition and dehydration. (18)

Cheryl Arenella, M.D., MPH, who has extensive experience in the field of Hospice and palliative care, offers the following examples of situations in which assisted nutrition and hydration are helpful to patients who are seriously ill:

- A person who has a mechanical blockage of his/her mouth, esophagus, or stomach, but is otherwise functioning fairly well, especially if this person is experiencing hunger, is likely to benefit if a tube is placed below the blockage in order to be able to receive nutrition and fluids. This is the case in many persons who suffer from head and neck or esophageal cancer, especially in the earlier stages of the cancer.
- In some cases, when a blocked bowel develops, such as in the spread of ovarian cancer, but the person is otherwise fairly functional, TPN (total parental nutrition) has been helpful in allowing that person to live and function longer than without the treatment.
- A person who has a temporary bout of severe nausea and vomiting or has diarrhea causing serious dehydration can often benefit from a short course of intravenous fluids to rest the bowel.
- Some persons with cachexia (a condition where the person keeps losing weight and does not eat well) due to HIV disease appear to benefit from assisted nutrition and hydration, especially those who have no active infection at the time of receiving it. (19)

On the other hand, there are cases in which assisted nutrition and hydration simply will not work and be effective in prolonging life. For example, a patient may be suffering from such severe heart, kidney, or liver failure that his body cannot process, metabolize, or excrete the nutrients or fluids supplied through the feeding device. (3) Or again, it may be virtually impossible to attach a feeding tube to a patient with nearly total body burn. (20) A feeding tube may not work because the tube itself has developed complications such as infection or bleeding, or because it has become entangled in the bowels so that the bowel tissue dies and can no longer absorb nutrients. (21) In such cases, assisted nutrition and hydration is a futile procedure in a very basic physiological sense (see chapter 6) and, according to the principle of weighing benefits and burdens, there is no moral obligation to use it.

Assisted nutrition and hydration also carries burdens of physical risks and complications. These have been enumerated by Dr. Cheryl Arenella:

- TPN (total parental nutrition) and central catheters can cause infection at the site of the catheter and in the catheter itself as well as sepsis (a generalized life-threatening infection). Pneumothorax (collapse of the lung) can occur at the time of inserting the catheter. Thrombosis (clots in the vein) can occur, causing local swelling. Sometimes these clots can travel to other parts of the body such as the brain or lung and can be life-threatening. Cardiac arrhythmias (irregularities of the heart beat) as well as electrolyte disturbances such as low sodium, low potassium or low blood sugar can occur. These are all potentially life-threatening.

- A nasogastric tube can cause choking and extreme discomfort at placement and afterwards. At the time of insertion, it can be misplaced in the trachea and cause pneumonia. The tube can cause erosions and abrasions, even perforations (holes) in the nasal passages, esophagus and stomach, and can cause acute and chronic bleeding. Aspiration pneumonia is a risk whenever an NG tube is in place. If a person is confused, he/she may need restraints to keep him/her from pulling the tube out. This can cause a whole host of problems, including psychic distress and increased agitation and anxiety, skin breakdown due to immobility, pneumonia due to immobility, and injury from restraints...
- A gastrostomy tube requires anesthesia during placement and has risks associated with the use of anesthesia. There is also a risk of infection of the abdominal wall and peritonitis (life threatening infection of the abdominal cavity). Gastrointestinal bleeding, blockage of the bowel or perforation of the bowel may occur. Diarrhea from the feeding formula is fairly common. Aspiration pneumonia is also common. If the person requires restraints to keep from pulling the tube out, the same complications listed above can occur.
- Intravenous fluids require IV tubing, with associated pain on insertion. Localized infection or cellulitis (a more serous infection of the skin that can spread) can occur. Thrombophlebitis (clotting in the vein) can occur and cause swelling and discomfort. Fluid overload is possible, causing swelling of the legs, arms and body. Electrolyte imbalances such as low sodium or low potassium are common. (19)

In sum, assisted nutrition and hydration is a mixed blessing. While it can benefit a patient, there are also definite burdens which can be associated with it. As with all treatments, decisions about using or forgoing assisted nutrition and hydration must be made on a case-by-case basis by considering the benefits and burdens of this procedure for a particular patient.

Common Misunderstandings about Assisted Nutrition and Hydration

The dietitian in our case study describes the removal of the feeding tube from Mrs. Ryan as "starving a patient to death." We often hear this phrase used in cases where a decision is made to withhold or withdraw assisted nutrition and hydration. But this description involves some misconceptions about forgoing assisted nutrition and hydration.

First, the phrase "starving a patient to death" carries the connotation that we are doing something to cause the patient's death, or engaging in an act of euthanasia. Second, the description "starving a patient to death" conjures up images of a painful, agonizing death.

One definition of euthanasia is "an action or an omission which of itself or by intention causes death, in order that all suffering may in this way be eliminated." (22) If we are dealing with some underlying fatal pathology which makes the assisted nutrition and hydration necessary in the first place (for example, a stroke which makes the patient unable to swallow), the removal or withholding of the feeding device merely allows that fatal pathology to take its natural course. It is the underlying fatal pathology, not the absence of assisted nutrition and hydration, that is the direct cause of death. Further, the intent behind the removal or withdrawal of assisted nutrition and hydration is important. If the purpose is one of intentionally ending the patient's life before death occurs naturally, then we are dealing with a case of euthanasia. On the other hand, if the purpose is to relieve the patient of a procedure that is of limited usefulness or unreasonably burdensome, then this decision can be seen as different than a decision to kill a patient. (18, 23) Thus withholding or withdrawing assisted nutrition and hydration under these conditions, namely, when an underlying fatal pathology directly causes death and the intent is to relieve the patient of a non-beneficial or very burdensome treatment, does not constitute an act of euthanasia on our part.

Second, the description "starving a patient to death" conjures up images of a painful, agonizing death. It is simply not true that a patient who is not given assisted nutrition and hydration will die in this way. For one thing, sensations of hunger and thirst can be relieved without using assisted nutrition and hydration. For example, ice chips or glycerin swabbing of the mouth can be used to relieve the thirst of dehydrated patients. (24, 25) Further, studies involving assisted nutrition and hydration for patients with varying degrees of consciousness have indicated that withdrawal of the feeding device does not cause suffering associated with hunger and dehydration. (14) Moreover, there is evidence that patients who are allowed to die without assisted nutrition and hydration may die more comfortably than patients who receive conventional amounts of intravenous hydration. (26) Dehydration can reduce swelling and increase comfort in a patient suffering from edema (swelling of the body caused by excess body fluids) or ascites (fluid in the abdominal cavity). Cough and congestion may be lessened because secretions in the lungs are diminished. A dehydrated person has less urine output so that problems with incontinence are lessened. Since there is less fluid in the gastrointestinal tract with dehydration, a patient may experience a decrease in nausea, vomiting, bloating, and regurgitation. Indeed, dehydration leads to death in ways that produce a sedative effect on the brain just before death, thus decreasing the need for pain medication. (19, 11, 25, 26) Consider the following actual case:

> David was a 64-year-old man with recurrent metastatic cancer of the larynx and tongue. Before being referred to the hospice program, he had received several years of therapy including surgery, radiation, and chemotherapy. He had massive facial and neck deformity with superimposed edema, which had resulted from treatment and recurrent disease. He had a continuous flow of secretions from the mouth and the tracheostomy site. His severe pain was managed with morphine sulfate, but maintaining his airway was a serious challenge. Although secretions could be removed by suctioning, the growing tumor and increasing edema threatened total airway occlusion.
>
> The patient, who was alert and oriented and had been feeding himself through a gastric tube, then decided to discontinue tube feedings. He lived 27 days after this decision. During that time, his appearance and comfort improved remarkably. Family members noted that the lessening facial edema made him look more like his usual self. The decrease in the neck edema resulted in a patent airway, which consequently eased the patient's breathing. A decrease in oral secretions also greatly added to his comfort. David remained mentally alert and interacted with his family. His pain was managed with approximately half of the morphine doses previously necessary. His death came quietly and comfortably. (27)

Providing food and water to a patient has been seen by some as a symbol of care and concern for that person. For this reason, they believe that tube feedings should always be provided to those who need it physically. But nutrition and hydration supplied by medical means is not always a good expression of loving care and concern:

> Food and water are certainly significant symbols, but the social experience associated with the giving and receiving of food and water may be

equally important. The patient receiving intravenous fluids, lying alone in a hospital bed, is having a much less rewarding experience than the patient in a personalized room being given ice chips by a concerned caregiver. Both are receiving water, but there are few other similarities. (28)

> Finally, what are the social and psychological effects of feeding techniques? With tube feedings, the caregiver may focus more attention on technical aspects, such as positioning the tube and checking the gastric residual, than on the patient. If feeding proceeds smoothly, contact between the patient and caregiver can be minimal. Moreover, the patient has no control over tube feedings except to pull out the tube. In contrast, during hand feedings the caregiver may be more attentive and affectionate, talking with the patient or holding his or her hand. Patients with few other ways of exercising control can still determine the timing, pace, and content of hand feeding. . . . Hand feedings that provide inadequate nutrition may meet more of the patient's needs than tube feedings that deliver adequate calories impersonally. The psychosocial effects of feeding techniques are especially important when the goal is supportive care. (29)

In sum, we must keep in mind that medical technologies can never replace personal presence and the human touch in caregiving.

For further discussion of assisted nutrition and hydration in the case of patients who are permanently unconscious, see chapter 9, "Treatment Decisions for PVS Patients."

Professional Association Guidelines

In working through difficult ethical dilemmas, health care workers can be assisted by guidelines developed by professional associations. In 1987 the American Dietetic Association published a position paper *Issues in Feeding the Terminally Ill Adult*. (25) According to this position paper, it is legitimate to forgo assisted nutrition and hydration in such cases when some or all of the following conditions are present:

- Death is imminent, within hours or a few days.
- Tube feeding will probably worsen the condition, symptoms, or pain, such as during shock, when pulmonary edema, vomiting, or aspiration would cause further complications.

- A competent patient has expressed an informed preference not to receive aggressive nutrition support which would be ineffective in improving the quality of life and/or which may be perceived by the patient as undignified, degrading, and physically or emotionally unacceptable.
- If available and legally recognized, written directives such as the "living will" or "durable power of attorney for medical care" may indicate the preference of an incompetent patient. Otherwise, the next of kin or guardian of an incompetent patient should be consulted about the patient's probable preference for the level of nutrition intervention. (25)

These guidelines are consistent with the ethical principles we have been using for making decisions about life-sustaining treatments (see chapter 6). The first and second bullet points fit with the principle of weighing benefits and burdens. The first bullet point can be interpreted as an application of the category of futile treatment, and the second bullet point deals with burdens which can be imposed on a patient by assisted nutrition and hydration. The third and fourth bullet points embody the concept of patient autonomy.

The American Dietetic Association subsequently released another position paper *Ethical and Legal Issues in Nutrition, Hydration, and Feeding*. (11) A section of this paper entitled "Suggested ethical deliberations about nutrition and hydration" contains the following points relevant to assisted nutrition and hydration:

1. The patient's expressed desire for extent of medical care is as primary guide for determining the level of nutrition intervention. . . .
3. The expected benefits, in contrast to the potential burdens, of nonoral feeding must be evaluated by the health care team and discussed with the patient. The focus of care should include the patient's physical and psychological comfort. . . .
5. Consider whether or not nutrition, either oral or artificial, will improve the patient's quality of life during the final stages of life.
6. Consider whether or not nutrient support, either oral or artificial, can be expected to provide the patient with emotional comfort, decreased anxiety about disease cachexia, improved self-esteem with cosmetic benefits, improved interpersonal relationships, or relief from fear of abandonment.
7. If death is imminent and feeding will not alter condition consider whether or not nutrient support will be burdensome. . . .
9. When tube feeding or parenteral feeding is being considered:
   a. The patient's informed preference for the level of nutritional intervention is primary. The patient or substitute decision maker should be advised on how to accomplish whatever feeding the patient desires.

b. When palliative care is the agreed goal nutritional support must be part of the palliative plan. A palliative care plan does not automatically preclude aggressive nutrition support. The decision to forgo "heroic" medical treatment does not preclude baseline nutrition support. All options for nutritional support can be considered.

c. Feeding may not be desirable if death is expected within hours or a few days and the effects of partial dehydration or the withdrawal of nutrition support will not adversely alter patient comfort. . . .

f. The potential benefits vs burdens of tube feeding or parenteral feeding should be weighed on the basis of specific facts concerning the patient's medical and mental status, as well as on the facility's options and limitations.

g. Facility options and limitations — One should consider the following:
  (1) Lack of staffing – no one to manage or monitor feeding
  (2) Too costly without financial help
  (3) If a feeding strategy is started on one site it will have to be stopped when the patient is transferred to another site, which can lead to a sense of abandonment. (11)

The position paper *Ethical and Legal Issues in Nutrition, Hydration, and Feeding* "affirms the patient's right to self-determination as the overriding principle." (11) This emphasis on patient autonomy is embodied in points 1 and 9a. However, the principle of weighing benefits and burdens is also invoked in points 3, 7, and 9f. In fact, points 6 and 9g can be interpreted as describing types of benefits and burdens to be taken into account.

This position paper likewise recognizes the role of an ethics committee in health care facilities. In recommending that "facilities should provide and distribute written protocols for the provision of and termination of tube feedings and parenteral feedings," it is mentioned that "the institution's ethics committee, if available, should assist in establishing and implementing defined, written guidelines for nutrition support protocol." (11) Or again, if a physician writes a diet order that the facility's registered dietitian does not agree with, "appeal to the facility's ethics mechanism (committee or consultant)" is advised. (11) Moreover, this position paper affirms that "registered dietitians should…serve as active members of institutional ethics committees." (11) Registered dietitians will bring to ethical discussions the technical knowledge of how to achieve desired feeding goals (11), and they "often have specific knowledge regarding the individual patient's preference because they discuss feeding issues with the patient and family." (11)

CHAPTER SUMMARY

Key Terms and Concepts

principle of patient autonomy: self-determination; the right of a patient to make the final decision in matters pertaining to his or her own life and health care.

principle of weighing benefits and burdens: It is morally permissible to forgo (that is, withhold or withdraw) a life-sustaining treatment if the burdens of the treatment outweigh its benefits or if the treatment is useless or futile.

Key Points

- The use of assisted nutrition and hydration on a short-term basis is not controversial. From an ethical point of view, what has been debated is the use of assisted nutrition and hydration for a prolonged period of time as a means (and sometimes the only means) of keeping a patient alive.
- Assisted nutrition and hydration has been variously categorized as standard nursing care, as medical treatment, as a natural, non-medical means of preserving life, and as a hybrid of medical treatment and basic health care.
- Procedures for providing assisted nutrition and hydration have burdens as well as benefits attached to them.
- Forgoing assisted nutrition and hydration in the presence of an underlying fatal pathology which directly causes death and with the intent of relieving the patient of a procedure that is of limited benefit or unreasonably burdensome, does *not* constitute an act of euthanasia.
- Comfort care can be provided to patients apart from using assisted nutrition and hydration. In fact, patients may die more comfortably without assisted nutrition and hydration than with it.
- Professional associations, such as the American Dietetic Association, have provided guidelines to assist health care providers in making decisions about using or forgoing assisted nutrition and hydration.

FOR FURTHER DISCUSSION

1. Consider the case of Barbara Ryan at the beginning of this chapter. Since dietitian Ron Kennedy disagrees with the decision to withdraw the

Chapter Eight

feeding tube from Barbara, he should, according to the American Dietetic Association, take his concerns to the ethics committee of the Forest Glen Nursing Home.

Role play this ethics consult. You will need participants to represent Barbara Ryan's daughter Ann, Barbara's son Robert, dietitian Ron Kennedy, and members of the ethics committee.

- What considerations is Ann likely to bring forward in support of removing the feeding tube from her mother? Do these arguments hold up?
- What is the dietitian Ron Kennedy likely to think and feel? What considerations might he raise against withdrawing the feeding tube? Do these arguments hold up?
- What ethical principles should be brought forward by members of the ethics committee? And how do these principles apply to Barbara's case?
- What ethical guidelines from the American Dietetic Association are relevant to this case?
- After listening to each point of view and considering the relevant ethical principles and guidelines, can the group reach agreement on what should be done in the case of Barbara Ryan?

2. Stephen Marshall, 67, has been fighting colon cancer for five years. He has undergone numerous rounds of chemotherapy. Initially, the chemotherapy seemed to stop the growth of the cancer, but in the last five months it has been ineffective. For this reason, Stephen has recently decided to discontinue the treatments. He tells his physician, Dr. Maria Garcia, that he is "ready to die" and just wants to be kept as comfortable as possible until that time comes. Dr. Garcia assures him that he will receive the best pain management available.

Stephen's condition continues to deteriorate. Because of the cancerous growth blocking his intestinal tract, Stephen cannot get adequate nutrition by normal means. Dr. Garcia asks Stephen if he wants a feeding tube placed. Dr. Garcia is honest in telling Stephen that the feeding tube will likely prolong his life—and his suffering—for a few months, at the most. Stephen tells Dr. Garcia that he doesn't want the feeding tube. A week later, Dr. Garcia again raises the issue of the feeding tube with Stephen just to be sure that Stephen hasn't changed his mind. Stephen indicates that he has discussed this matter with his wife Patricia, and that she supports him in his decision to refuse the feeding tube. Dr. Garcia does not bring up the issue again. Stephen begins hospice care at home.

When Stephen and Patricia's adult daughter Alice comes to visit, she feels uncomfortable that a feeding tube is not being used for her father. Alice says that she can understand withholding a feeding tube from a dying person who is "out of it" and doesn't know what is going on. However, she states that she can't deal with withholding feeding from someone who is mentally alert—like her father—and talks to her when she comes into his room.

Alice is deeply concerned about her father, and decides to contact Roberta Summers, a high school classmate who now works as a registered dietitian at the local community hospital and serves on its ethics committee. Alice and Roberta make arrangements to meet for lunch to discuss the situation.

Suppose you are the registered dietitian Roberta Summers. What would you say to Alice about using/forgoing a feeding tube for her father? As a member of a health care ethics committee, what ethical principles might you bring into the discussion? Are any ethical guidelines from your professional association, the American Dietetic Association, of help in determining the right thing to do?

You might want to role play the conversation between Alice and Roberta.

References

1. Gregory E. Pence, *Classic Cases in Medical Ethics,* 2nd ed. (New York: McGraw-Hill, 1995), chap. 1.
2. David Major, M.D., "The Medical Procedures for Providing Food and Water: Indications and Effects" in Joanne Lynn (ed.), *By No Extraordinary Means: The Choice to Forgo Life-Sustaining Food and Water* (Bloomington, IN: Indiana University Press, 1986).
3. Myles Sheehan, S.J., M.D., ""Feeding Tubes: Sorting Out the Issues," *Health Progress* 82/6 (Nov.-Dec. 2001): 22-7.
4. Gilbert Meilaender, "On Removing Food and Water: Against the Stream," *Hastings Center Report* 14/6 (December 1984): 11-13.
5. New Jersey State Catholic Conference, "Providing Food and Fluids to Severely Brain Damaged Patients," *Origins* 16/32 (Jan. 22, 1987): 582-84.
6. Patrick G. Derr, "Nutrition and Hydration as Elective Therapy: Brophy and Jobes from an Ethical and Historical Perspective," *Issues in Law & Medicine* 2/1 (1986): 25-38.
7. Patrick G. Derr, "Why Food and Fluids Can Never Be Denied," *Hastings Center Report* 16/1 (February 1986): 28-30.
8. Dennis Brodeur, "Is a Decision to Forgo Tube Feeding for Another a Decision to Kill?," *Issues in Law and Medicine* 6/4 (1991): 395-406.

9. American Academy of Neurology, "Position of the American Academy of Neurology on Certain Aspects of the Care and Management of the Pesistent Vegetative State Patient," *Neurology* 39 (January 1989): 125-26, reprinted in James J. Walter & Thomas A. Shannon (eds.), *Quality of Life: The New Medical Dilemma* (New York: Paulist Press, 1990).
10. *Cruzan v. Director, Missouri Department of Health*, 110 S. Ct. 2841 (1990).
11. American Dietetic Association, "Position of the American Dietetic Association: Ethical and Legal Issues in Nutrition, Hydration, and Feeding," *Journal of the American Dietetic Association* 108 (2008): 873-82.
12. John Paul II, "Care for Patients in a 'Permanent' Vegetative State," *Origins* 33/43 (April 8, 2004): 737-40.
13. Congregation for the Doctrine of the Faith, Commentary on *Responses to Certain Questions of the United States Conference of Catholic Bishops Concerning Artificial Nutrition and Hydration* (August 1, 2007), http://www.vatican.va> Holy See English > Roman Curia > Congregations > Doctrine of the Faith > Doctrinal Documents. Accessed January 2009.
14. Dan O'Brien, John Paul Slosar, and Anthony R. Tersigni, "Utilitarian Pessimism, Human Dignity, and the Vegetative State A Practical Analysis of the Papal Allocution," *The National Catholic Bioethics Quarterly* 4/3 (Autumn 2004): 497-512.
15. Kevin D. O'Rourke, O.P., "The Catholic Tradition on Forgoing Life Support," *The National Catholic Bioethics Quarterly* 5/3 (Autumn 2005): 537-53.
16. Bishops Committee on Doctrine and Morals (Australian Catholic Bishops' Conference), Bishops Committee for Health Care (Australia), and Catholic Health Australia, "Briefing Note on the Obligation to Provide Nutrition and Hydration" (September 3, 2004), http://www.acbc.catholic.org.au/bc/docmoral/ articlelist2004.htm or http://www.cha.org.au/site.php?id=666. Accessed January 2009.
17. Bernard Lo & Laurie Dornbrand, "Understanding the Benefits and Burdens of Tube Feedings," *Archives of Internal Medicine* 149/9 (September 1989): 1925-6.
18. Pikes Peak Forum for Health Care, *Decisions About the End of Life... Help for Those Who Must Decide* (March 2008), http://www.pikespeakforum.org/PDF/PPFHCbookletMar2008.pdf. Accessed January 2009.
19. Cheryl Arenella, "Artificial Nutrition and Hydration: Beneficial or Harmful?" (2005), http://www.americanhospice.org/index.php?option=com_content&task=view&id=48&Itemid=8. Accessed January 2009.

20. Joanne Lynn & James F. Childress, "Must Patients Always Be Given Food and Water?" in Joanne Lynn (ed.), *By No Extraordinary Means: The Choice to Forgo Life-Sustaining Food and Water* (Bloomington, IN: Indiana University Press, 1986).
21. Daniel P. Sulmasy, "Preserving Life? The Vatican & PVS," *Commonweal* 134/21 (Dec. 7, 2007): 16-18.
22. Congregation for the Doctrine of the Faith, *Declaration on Euthanasia* (Washington, DC: United States Catholic Conference, 1980).
23. Committee for Pro-Life Activities of the National Conference of Catholic Bishops, "Nutrition and Hydration: Moral and Pastoral Reflections," *Origins* 21/44 (April 9, 1992): 705-12.
24. Hastings Center, *Guidelines on the Termination of Life-Sustaining Treatment and the Care of the Dying* (Briarcliff Manor, NY: Hastings Center, 1987).
25. American Dietetic Association, "Position of the American Dietetic Association: Issues in Feeding the Terminally Ill Adult," *American Dietetic Association Journal* 87 (January-April 1987): 78-85.
26. Joyce C. Zerwekh, "The Dehydration Question," Nursing 83 (January 1983): 47-51.
27. Shirley Ann Smith, "Controversies in Hydrating the Terminally Ill Patient," *Journal of Intravenous Nursing* 20/4 (July/August 1997): 193-200.
28. Phyllis Schmitz and Merry O'Brien, "Observations on Nutrition and Hydration in Dying Cancer Patients" in Joanne Lynn (ed.), *By No Extraordinary Means: The Choice to Forgo Life-Sustaining Food and Water* (Bloomington, IN: Indiana University Press, 1986).
29. Bernard Lo and Laurie Dornbrand, "Guiding the Hand that Feeds: Caring for the Demented Elderly," *New England Journal of Medicine* 311/6 (August 9, 1984): 402-4.

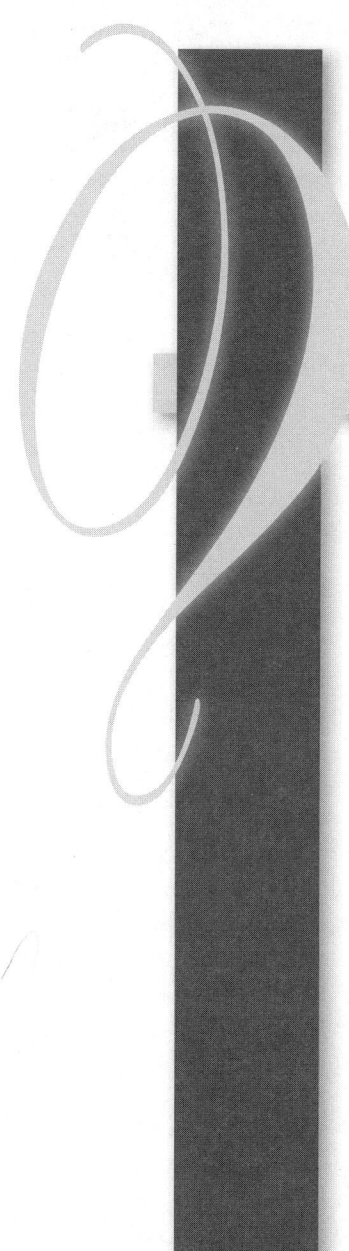

Chapter 9

Treatment Decisions for Vegetative State Patients

Three highly publicized court cases concerning the withdrawal of life-sustaining treatments have involved young adult women: Karen Ann Quinlan, Nancy Cruzan, and Terri Schiavo. In the case of Karen Ann Quinlan, at issue was the removal of a ventilator. In the cases of Nancy Cruzan and Terri Schiavo, the removal of a feeding tube proved controversial. What these women shared in common was a diagnosis of being in a permanent vegetative state. (1)

In this chapter you will learn:

- medical facts about the vegetative state;
- treatment options for patients in this condition;
- how the principle of autonomy and the principle of weighing benefits and burdens apply to treatment decisions for vegetative state patients;

- what special ethical issues arise in making treatment decisions for these patients;
- guidelines of a professional association for providing assisted nutrition and hydration to vegetative state patients.

Case Study

Donald Pollack, 35, and Louise Caldwell, 32, have been married for six years. They have two children, Jessica, 4, and Eric, 2. All her life Louise has had heart problems because of a congenital heart defect. She feels very fortunate to have been able to carry the two children she now has. Both Don and Louise have established careers as attorneys.

Late one afternoon, a neighbor finds Louise lying on the front porch of her home. Apparently, Louise had stopped at home on her way to pick up her children at the day care center when something happened to her. The neighbor calls 911. The paramedics who arrive tell the neighbor that Louise has suffered a cardiac arrest. CPR is administered to restore her heartbeat, and she is taken to the emergency room of the local hospital.

When her husband Don arrives at the hospital, he finds that Louise has been put in the intensive care unit (ICU) and placed on a ventilator. Three weeks go by, and Louise remains "out of it." There are periods of time when her eyes are open but she doesn't seem aware of anyone in the room. She doesn't speak, and when the doctor tries to get her to respond to simple commands, she doesn't. She is now able to be taken off the ventilator and can breathe on her own, but she must be fed through a tube. A neurologist who examines Louise diagnoses her as being in a "vegetative state."

Louise is transferred to the Woodlands Care Center. Her care at the nursing home includes tube feeding, maintaining skin care and appropriate hygiene, range of motion exercises to minimize limb contracture, and time sitting out of bed.

A month after admission to the Woodlands Care Center—and seven weeks after the cardiac arrest that put her in this condition—Louise develops pneumonia. She is again examined by a neurologist, who tells Don that his wife is now in a "persistent vegetative state" and that he will have to make decisions about the kinds of treatments which should and should not be provided for his wife.

Without hesitation, Don insists that antibiotics—and any other treatment medically indicated—be provided for his wife. It is too soon, he believes, to

> give up on the possibility of his wife's recovery. He himself has seen several cases of patients who were written off as "hopeless" by doctors but who eventually recovered. Besides, he points out that his wife is still young, only 32 years old—much too young to be allowed to die. Indeed, for the sake of their two young children who need a mother, Don wants "everything possible" done to save Louise.
>
> John Miller is the physical therapist supervising Louise's range of motion exercises. He personally is glad that Louise's husband has made this decision. After all, how could health care professionals let someone die whose eyes are open?
>
> ■ ■ ■

Medical Facts about the Vegetative State

Before considering the ethical issues surrounding care of vegetative state patients, it is very important to know certain medical facts about this condition. The term "persistent vegetative state" (abbreviated as PVS) has often been used generically. More technically, a distinction is made between a vegetative state, a *persistent* vegetative state, and a *permanent* vegetative state. (2, 3)

A *vegetative state* is one form of unconsciousness. It is deceptive to observers because the patient goes through sleep-wake cycles so that there are times when the patient's eyes are open. However, there is no indication that the patient is aware of herself or the environment. Some brain functions are still intact either completely or partially; namely, those controlled by the hypothalamus and the brain stem. (2)

A task force sponsored by five different American medical societies has proposed the following criteria for diagnosing a vegetative state:

- The patient gives no evidence of being aware of self or the environment, and is unable to interact with others.
- The patient gives no evidence of sustained, reproducible, purposeful, or voluntary behavioral responses to stimuli.
- The patient gives no evidence of understanding or using language.
- The patient goes through sleep-wake cycles.
- The brain functions of the hypothalamus and brain stem are sufficiently preserved to allow the patient to survive with medical and nursing care.

- The patient has incontinence of both bowel and bladder.
- Cranial-nerve reflexes (e.g., reaction of the pupils to light, the gag reflex) and spinal reflexes are preserved in varying degrees. (2, 3)

A patient in a vegetative state may occasionally grunt, scream, smile, or shed tears, and show movement of nonparalyzed limbs. Again, this can be deceiving to observers, who mistakenly take this activity as a sign of consciousness. (2, 3)

A *persistent vegetative state* is defined as a vegetative state which has continued for at least one month. It can occur after an acute traumatic brain injury (e.g., an injury due to a car accident) or after an acute nontraumatic brain injury (e.g., cardiac arrest). It can be caused by degenerative or metabolic disorders (e.g., Alzheimer's disease, Parkinson's disease, Huntington's disease) or by developmental malformations in infants and children (e.g., anencephalic infants in whom part of the brain never develops). (2, 3) Sometimes a patient in a persistent vegetative state because of an acute traumatic or nontraumatic brain injury will regain consciousness and abilities to function in various ways, but the probabilities of this happening are not particularly high. (4)

A patient in a persistent vegetative state is said to enter a *permanent vegetative state* when the diagnosis is that the condition is irreversible and the chance that the patient will regain consciousness is very, very small. (2, 3) In the case of a traumatic brain injury, a persistent vegetative state can be considered permanent twelve months after the injury in both adults and children. Recovery after this time is very rare, and almost always involves severe disability. If the persistent vegetative state is related to a nontraumatic injury, it can be considered permanent after three months in both adults and children. While recovery does occur after this time period, it is rare and involves moderate or severe disability. (4) Patients who are in a vegetative state due to degenerative or metabolic diseases have no possibility of recovery. (4) For infants and children with brain malformations severe enough to cause developmental vegetative states, lack of consciousness by the age of six months almost completely precludes the potential for future improvement. (4) In the case of anencephalic infants, it is clear at birth that there is no possibility for recovery because the complete absence of the cerebral cortex of the brain precludes consciousness. (4)

The term "vegetative state" was chosen to name the condition in question because "*to vegetate* is defined in the Oxford English dictionary as 'to live a merely physical life, devoid of intellectual activity or social intercourse (1740)' and *vegetative* is used to describe 'an organic body capable of growth and development but devoid of sensation and thought (1764)'." (5) However, some have taken this terminology in a pejorative sense, prompting affirmations that a human being, "*even if seriously ill or disabled in the exercise of his highest functions, is and always will be a man*, and he will never become a 'vegetable' or an 'animal'."(6) Concomitantly, it is affirmed that "the intrinsic value and personal dignity of every human being do not change, no matter what the concrete circumstances of his or her life." (6) Thus some have substituted the term "post-coma unresponsive" for "vegetative state." (7) Following the medical literature, we will use the term "vegetative state," understanding that the use of this term is not intended to carry a negative connotation about the human status and dignity of patients in this condition.

A vegetative state is different from a *coma*. In a coma, a patient's eyes remain closed, and the person appears to be asleep but cannot be aroused. (2, 3) The patient does not go through sleep-wake cycles as happens in the vegetative state. (3) A vegetative state has also been distinguished from a *minimally conscious state*, "a condition of severely altered consciousness in which minimal but definite behavioral evidence of self or environmental awareness is demonstrated." (8) A vegetative state should not be confused with *locked-in syndrome*, "a rare neurological disorder characterized by complete paralysis of voluntary muscles in all parts of the body except for those that control eye movements." (9) Individuals suffering from this disorder "are conscious and can think and reason, but are unable to speak or move." (9)

Most patients in a persistent or permanent vegetative state who survive for a long time are able to breathe on their own and have a functioning cardiovascular system. (2) While most vegetative state patients show some response to painful stimuli (e.g., limb withdrawal, facial grimacing, groaning, rise in respiratory and pulse rates and blood pressure), it is "generally held that these responses are all at reflex level and do not indicate that pain is being experienced at a conscious level." (5) That vegetative state patients do not *experience* pain or suffering is reinforced by the fact of depression of the cerebral metabolic rate for glucose to levels equivalent to deep surgical anesthesia in vegetative patients. (5) This claim is also reinforced by the fact that "pathological examination shows such extensive bilateral damage to the cerebral hemispheres or their connections with the thalamus that the structural mechanisms for such experiences are no longer available." (5)

Because of the severe brain injury necessary to produce the vegetative state, the average life expectancy of such patients is two to five years. (4) However, a very small number of patients "have survived for more than 15 years . . . including three patients who survived for more than 17, 37, and 41 years." (4) Reported causes of death for patients in a persistent or permanent vegetative state include pulmonary or urinary tract infection, generalized systemic failure, respiratory failure, and recurrent strokes or tumors. (4)

The ethical controversy over using or forgoing treatments for vegetative state patients has focused on those who have reached the stage of being in a persistent or permanent vegetative state, and most especially, those in a permanent vegetative state. Thus these patients will be the focus of our discussion.

Treatment Decisions for Vegetative State Patients

A patient in a persistent or permanent vegetative state needs various kinds of care:

> Preventive care is foremost. Daily exercises in a range of movements slow the formation of limb contractures, which otherwise become particularly severe in patients in a persistent vegetative state. Daily skin care and frequent repositioning of the patient prevent decubitus ulcers. A tracheostomy may be required to maintain airway patency and prevent aspiration pneumonia. Bladder and bowel care is desirable for hygienic reasons. Since pulmonary and urinary tract infections are common, appropriate monitoring and, if necessary, treatment with antibiotics are required. Placement of nasogastric, gastrostomy, or jejunostomy feeding tubes is usually necessary to maintain adequate nutrition and hydration. (4)

Those responsible for making health care decisions for persistent and permanent vegetative state patients are faced with choosing among several possible levels of treatment:

- Continue routine nursing care, but stop all treatments necessary for prolonging life, including assisted nutrition and hydration.
- Continue assisted nutrition and hydration as well as routine nursing care, but do not add any additional procedures or treatments.
- Continue assisted nutrition and hydration as well as routine nursing care, and in addition add procedures or treatments such as the following if they become necessary for prolonging life: antibiotics, simple diagnostic tests, blood or blood product transfusions, transfer to the intensive care unit (ICU), dialysis, chemotherapy for cancer, minor surgery, major surgery, mechanical ventilation, cardiopulmonary resuscitation, organ transplantation. (4, 10)

For example, in the case study above, Louise's husband Don has decided that he wants everything provided that is needed medically by his wife (e.g., antibiotics as well as tube feeding).

A patient who is in a persistent or permanent vegetative state is not capable of making decisions, so that a proxy must make decisions on her behalf. The preferred standard for proxy decision making is the *principle of substituted judgment,* which directs the proxy to make treatment decisions in accord with directives explicitly given by the patient or, lacking these, in accord with the beliefs, values, preferences, and life-long behavior patterns of the patient. This method of proxy decision making is regarded as an extension of *patient autonomy.* (See chapter 7, "Proxy Decision Making and Advance Directives.") However, a patient's own autonomous judgment, as well as a proxy's substituted judgment, ought to be guided by the *principle of weighing benefits and burdens.* Thus, the proxy should ask: How would this patient judge the respective benefits and burdens of a certain treatment administered while in a persistent or permanent vegetative state? (See chapter 6, "Making Decisions about Using or Forgoing Life-Sustaining Treatments.")

Some would say that the basic purpose of using treatments to prolong the life of a vegetative state patient is to enable the patient to survive long enough to recover consciousness and function. This possible recovery is seen as the benefit of the life-sustaining treatments. Hence, when a patient is diagnosed as being in a permanent vegetative state, this benefit of using life-sustaining treatments is very, very unlikely to occur. According to this point of view, treatment decisions for someone in a permanent vegetative state may be different from decisions for someone in a persistent vegetative state where recovery is still a possibility. (11)

Consider the case study involving Louise. She has been in a vegetative state for over one month (specifically, for seven weeks) so that she can be reliably diagnosed as being in a *persistent* vegetative state. Her condition is due to a nontraumatic injury (a cardiac arrest), and studies indicate that three months must elapse before her vegetative condition can be judged to be permanent. However, studies also indicate that when a persistent vegetative state is due to a nontraumatic injury, only 11 percent of such patients recover consciousness by three months after the injury. (4)

In Louise's case, there is still some chance (although not great) that life-prolonging treatments will make possible the benefit of recovering consciousness. If Louise's husband Don believes that she would want to take this chance, then it is appropriate for him to want life-sustaining treatments to be used at the present time. However, if Louise does not regain consciousness but her condition progresses into a permanent vegetative state, then assessment about the value of providing treatments may change.

Further, it should be kept in mind that a patient in a persistent or permanent vegetative state could experience problems that qualify as *burdensome* aspects of continued treatment. For example, such patients are susceptible to feeding-tube site infections, incontinence and other bowel and bladder disorders, bedsores, and deformities caused by muscle deterioration and contracture. These are genuine burdens for the patient even if the patient does not consciously experience them. (12)

Particularly controversial has been the withdrawal of assisted nutrition and hydration from patients in a persistent or permanent vegetative state. According to the principle of weighing benefits and burdens (see chapter 6, "Making Decisions about Using or Forgoing Life-Sustaining Treatments"), such withdrawal is permissible if assisted nutrition and hydration proves useless or futile, providing no benefit to the patient, or if it proves more burdensome than beneficial. Thus the principle of weighing benefits and burdens would justify withdrawing assisted nutrition and hydration from a patient in a persistent or permanent vegetative state if the feeding tube does not work because the tube itself has developed complications such as infection or bleeding, or because it has become tangled in the bowels so that the bowel tissue dies and can no longer absorb nutrients. (13) Or again, this ethical principle could justify withdrawing assisted nutrition and hydration on grounds of excessive burdens if the vegetative state patient experiences recurrent pneumonia caused by feedings going up the food pipe and down the windpipe. (13) The same would hold true if the feeding tube is involved in complications such as causing diarrhea that has resulted in infected ulcers, or causing electrolyte abnormalities that has led to seizures. (13)

When artificial nutrition and hydration are withdrawn, patients in a persistent or permanent vegetative state usually die within ten to fourteen days. Dehydration and electrolyte imbalance, rather than malnutrition, are the immediate causes of death. Except for dryness of the skin and mucous membranes, it is not readily apparent to family members that the patient is dying of dehydration. Further, appropriate nursing care can prevent these signs of dehydration. Facial swelling can occur as a result of prolonged administration of artificial nutrition and hydration but, as the patient becomes dehydrated, this swelling decreases and facial features may assume a more normal appearance during the last few days of life. (4) Some fear that allowing persistent or permanent vegetative state patients to die in this way is condemning them to an excruciatingly painful death. Thus the aforementioned evidence that vegetative state patients do not *experience* pain or suffering is important.

Special Ethical Questions in Treatment Decisions for Vegetative State Patients

One issue in the debate over how to treat patients in a persistent or permanent vegetative state is whether such patients should be regarded as *disabled* or as *dying.* (14, 15, 16, 17) From a moral point of view, this is not a trivial question. If one judges that the persistent or permanent vegetative state is a disability, then all the concern and help we offer to disabled and handicapped persons should be given to persons in this condition; consideration of forgoing life-sustaining treatments becomes inappropriate.

Those who take the position that a patient in a persistent or permanent vegetative state is "disabled but not dying" point out that such a patient can often have her life prolonged for months or even years through assisted nutrition and hydration. Hence, we are not dealing with a situation in which inevitable death is imminent. (18)

On the other hand, it can be argued that the persistent or permanent vegetative state qualifies as a fatal pathology since this condition involves serious damage or malformation in the brain. The brain is the "integrating organ of the entire person" and "severe trauma to the brain . . . generally causes various medical problems that can accurately be described as pathologies." (19) Moreover, it is argued that, even if the persistent or permanent vegetative state is not technically "terminal" (defined as a condition from which a person is likely to die in a short time regardless of what treatments are applied), this state still qualifies as a "lethal" condition since the patient will die of this condition unless treatment is given. (20)

Another issue in the debate over how to treat patients in a persistent or permanent vegetative state is the value of prolonging life on a merely biological level. While certain bodily functions are retained, such patients have lost consciousness and all the accompanying abilities which, most of all, seem to make us human:

> Most of what makes someone a distinctive individual is lost when the person is unconscious, especially if he or she will always remain so. Personality, memory, purposive action, social interaction, sentience, thought, and even emotional states are gone. Only vegetative functions and reflexes persist. If food is supplied, the digestive system functions and uncontrolled evacuation occurs; the kidneys produce urine; the heart, lungs, and blood vessels continue to move air and blood; and nutrients are distributed in the body. (21)

It is a matter of debate whether the prolongation of mere biological function is a benefit to a person, and a benefit sufficient to justify the use of life-sustaining treatments. Some argue that "human bodily life is a great good" and in fact that "such life is inherently good, not merely instrumental to other goods." (16) Others contend that medicine is about "human wholeness," a wholeness which "means a certain well-working of the enlivened body and its unimpaired powers to sense, think, feel, desire, move, and maintain itself. . . ." (22)

In sum, if one believes that biological life is valuable in and of itself, then one will likely regard life-sustaining treatments as providing a benefit even to patients in a permanent vegetative state. One the other hand, if one believes that it is mental activities that are most truly human and that bodily health is a means to this end, then one is not likely to see the use of life-sustaining treatments as beneficial to such patients.

Our medical resources are limited. Another issue that has arisen in the care of patients in a persistent, and especially, those in a permanent vegetative state concerns the *allocation of medical resources*. As a society, should we use our medical resources to sustain the lives of such patients when these same resources could be used for other patients who would be judged to benefit more? This question was raised (and answered in the negative) by a presidential commission on bioethical issues:

> An irresponsible stewardship of society's resources can occur when a permanently unconscious patient is given care that precludes the treatment of others who would be helped far more than the unconscious patient. This could occur, for example, were another patient to receive less beneficial therapy because a scarce support system is being used with a permanently unconscious patient. Whenever there is reason to believe this is happening, the patient with a remediable illness or even a chance of regaining consciousness should be put on the support system even if it precipitates the death of the permanently unconscious patient. . . .
>
> A second failure of responsible stewardship occurs when resources are expended so lavishly in the care of patients who will never regain consciousness that other important social goals are thwarted. . . . since it is ethically acceptable to limit the provision of treatment, especially when it can at best offer a very small benefit to the patient, policymakers in public and private health care payment programs may legitimately consider means of limiting, or even proscribing, these expenditures. (21)

Ethically, this issue involves distributive justice, or fairness in the distribution of benefits, burdens, and resources (see chapter 1). The value one places (or does not place) on sustaining life on a purely biological level will affect how one judges the use of medical resources for persistent and permanent vegetative state patients (and whether one disagrees or agrees with the recommendations of the presidential commission).

Guidelines from a Professional Association

As already noted, the issue of providing assisted nutrition and hydration to vegetative state patients has been especially controversial. The American Dietetic Association (ADA) formulated guidelines for feeding such patients.

- Feeding should start for a patient in a coma or an unconscious state as soon as he or she is medically stable and should continue at least until a diagnosis of PVS is established.
- Feeding should only be stopped after the patient is diagnosed as permanently unconscious and there is evidence of the patient's wish to stop nutrition and hydration. (23)

It should be noted that there are two conditions placed on stopping assisted nutrition and hydration. In addition to the state of unconsciousness being diagnosed as permanent, it must be the case that the patient herself would not want nutrition and hydration in such a condition. The second condition is emphasized in the ADA's position paper:

> Guidelines for feeding a permanently unconscious patient support the patient's right to self-determination as the overriding principle. Within American society, the individual's right to self-determination generally takes precedence over the beliefs or wishes of health care providers.
>
> The patient's expressed desire is the primary guide for determining the extent of nutrition and hydration once the patient is diagnosed as being in a PVS.

From an ethical point of view, the American Dietetic Association is placing a premium on patient autonomy.

CHAPTER SUMMARY

Key Terms and Concepts

vegetative state: one form of unconsciousness in which the patient goes through sleep-wake cycles but has no awareness of self or the environment.
persistent vegetative state: a vegetative state that has continued for at least one month.

permanent vegetative state: a vegetative state that is most likely irreversible.
principle of patient autonomy: self-determination; the right of a patient to make the final decision in matters pertaining to his or her own life and health care.
principle of substituted judgment: a proxy decision maker attempts to reach the decision that the patient would make if he or she were able to choose, relying on written or oral directives explicitly given by the patient or on knowledge of the patient's beliefs, values, preferences, and life-long behavior patterns.
principle of weighing benefits and burdens: it is morally permissible to forgo (that is, withhold or withdraw) a life-sustaining treatment if the burdens of the treatment outweigh its benefits or if the treatment is useless or futile, providing no benefit to the patient.
principle of distributive justice: an ethical principle concerning fairness in the distribution of benefits, burdens, and resources.

Key Points

- A patient in a persistent or permanent vegetative state needs routine nursing care (for example, skin care, repositioning, bladder and bowel care). In addition, treatment decisions will have to be made about using or forgoing assisted nutrition and hydration (tube feeding), and perhaps about such treatments and procedures as antibiotics, diagnostic tests, blood or blood product transfusions, transfer to the ICU, dialysis, chemotherapy, surgery, ventilators, and resuscitation.
- In making these treatment decisions, the proxy decision maker should consider what the patient herself would want done (principle of patient autonomy) in view of the benefits and burdens of the treatments.
- There are cases in which the principle of weighing benefits and burdens justifies forgoing treatments, including assisted nutrition and hydration, in the case of the vegetative state patient.
- According to one point of view, the intended benefit of keeping someone alive in a vegetative state is to allow for the possibility of recovery of consciousness and function. Hence, it may be reasonable to make different decisions about the use of life-sustaining treatments when the patient is diagnosed as being in a permanent vegetative state than when the patient is first diagnosed as being in a persistent vegetative state.

- One point of controversy about treatment decisions for patients in a persistent or permanent vegetative state is whether such a patient is merely disabled or dying.
- Another point of controversy involves a judgment about the value of prolonging life on a biological level without mental function.
- Yet another issue concerns the just allocation of medical resources among patients at individual and societal levels.

FOR FURTHER DISCUSSION

Suppose that you are the allied health representative on your facility's ethics committee, and that the following cases involving vegetative state patients are brought to the committee for an ethics consult. In making a recommendation for care, the following options are available:

1. Continue routine nursing care, but stop all treatments necessary for prolonging life, including assisted nutrition and hydration.
2. Continue assisted nutrition and hydration as well as routine nursing care, but do not add any additional procedures or treatments.
3. Continue assisted nutrition and hydration as well as routine nursing care, and in addition add (some or all of) such treatments as the following if they become necessary for prolonging life: antibiotics, simple diagnostic tests, blood or blood product transfusions, transfer to the intensive care unit, dialysis, chemotherapy for cancer, minor surgery, major surgery, mechanical ventilation, cardiopulmonary resuscitation, organ transplantation.
4. Other (describe).

Case 1. Patricia Farrell, 33, has been diagnosed as being in a permanent vegetative state. Since she became unconscious after a car accident fifteen months ago, Patricia has been on assisted nutrition and hydration. Recently she has developed aspiration pneumonia from the feeding tube. Patricia's physician, Dr. Eileen Swanson, speaks with her husband, Richard, and recommends against the use of antibiotics. Indeed, Dr. Swanson mentions to Richard that perhaps it is time to think about removing the feeding tube as well. Richard, however, insists that the doctor "do everything" to save his wife. Richard admits that, after the death of her father, Patricia had stated quite clearly that she herself wanted to "go quickly" and did not wish to linger on for several years in a debilitated state, as had happened to her father. Nevertheless, Richard says that "miracles can happen," and that he just doesn't feel right about "giving up" on Patricia at this point. Richard says that he would feel guilty that he would be doing something to "kill" his wife in consenting to withdrawal of the feeding tube. Because Dr. Swanson is concerned that Richard has false hopes for his wife, she encourages him to meet with the facility's ethics committee to talk about the situation.

Case 2. Consider again the case of Patricia Farrell, with the following change of circumstances: Richard relates that, after the death of her father, Patricia had stated quite clearly that, if anything happened to her so that she could not take care of herself, she did not want anything done to shorten or prematurely take her life, as she believed had happened to her father while in the hospital.

Case 3. Two months ago Tom McGann, 45, suffered a serious a brain injury in a car accident. Since that time he has been unconscious, and a neurologist has told his wife, Alice, that he is in a persistent vegetative state. Assisted nutrition and hydration has been used during this time to sustain his life. Tom has recently developed kidney problems, and Alice must now make a decision about dialysis. Tom had always been very active physically, golfing, bowling, and taking long bicycle rides on nature trails. Because of this, Alice feels that Tom would never want to continue to exist in an unconscious state, confined to bed, and not able to do any of the things he enjoyed about life. Kidney failure, Alice believes, may be a blessing in disguise, "letting her husband go free." Alice tells her husband's doctor that dialysis should not be started. However, because this decision will ensure that Tom will die, the doctor encourages Alice to talk with the facility's ethics committee before she makes the final decision.

First, go through each scenario on your own. Decide on your recommendation. Write a brief explanation of the factors and ethical principles you considered in deciding on that course of action. Share and discuss your recommendations with other members of the class (as you would with other members of the ethics committee on which you serve). This may be done either in small groups or with the class as a whole. Can you reach agreement about what ought to be done in each of the various case scenarios?

References

1. Gregory E. Pence, *Classic Cases in Medical Ethics*, 5th ed. (New York: McGraw-Hill, 2007).
2. The Multi-Society Task Force on PVS, "Medical Aspects of the Persistent Vegetative State," Part One, *New England Journal of Medicine* 330/21 (May 26, 1994):1499-1508.
3. American Neurological Association Committee on Ethical Affairs, "Persistent Vegetative State: Report of the American Neurological Association Committee on Ethical Affairs," *Annals of Neurology* 33/4 (April 1993): 386-90.
4. Multi-Society Task Force on PVS, "Medical Aspects of the Persistent Vegetative State," Part Two, *New England Journal of Medicine* 330/22 (June 2, 1994): 1572-79.
5. Bryan Jennett, *The Vegetative State Medical facts, ethical and legal dilemmas* (New York: Cambridge University Press, 2002).
6. Pope John Paul II, "To the Participants in the International Congress on 'Life-Sustaining Treatments and Vegetative State: Scientific Advances and Ethical Dilemmas'," in Arthur L. Caplan, James J. McCartney, and Dominic A. Sisti, *The Case of Terri Schiavo Ethics at the End of Life* (Amherst, NY: Prometheus Books, 2006).
7. Bishops Committee on Doctrine and Morals (Australian Catholic Bishops' Conference), Bishops Committee for Health Care (Australia), and Catholic Health Australia, "Briefing Note on the Obligation to Provide Nutrition and Hydration" (September 3, 2004), http://www.acbc.catholic.org.au/bc/docmoral/articlelist2004.htm or http://www.cha.org.au/site.php?id=666. Accessed January 2009.
8. J.T. Giacino, S. Ashwal, N. Childs, R. Cranford, B. Jennett, D.I. Katz, J.P. Kelly, J.H. Rosenberg, J. Whyte, R.D. Zafonte, and N.D. Zasler, "The minimally conscious state Definition and diagnostic criteria," *Neurology* 58/3 (Feb. 2002): 349-53.
9. National Institute of Neurological Disorders and Stroke, National Institutes of Health, *Locked-in Syndrome Information Page*. http://www.ninds.nih.gov/disorders/lockedinsyndrome/lockedinsyndrome.htm Accessed February 2009.
10. Ellen Fox and Carol Stocking, "Ethics Consultants' Recommendations for Life-Prolonging Treatment of Patients in a Persistent Vegetative State," *Journal of the American Medical Association* 270/21 (December 1, 1993): 2578-82.
11. American Academy of Neurology, "Position of the American Academy of Neurology on Certain Aspects of the Care and Management of the

Persistent Vegetative State Patient," *Neurology* 39 (January 1989): 125-26, reprinted in James J. Walter & Thomas A. Shannon (eds.), *Quality of Life The New Medical Dilemma* (New York: Paulist Press, 1990).

12. Michael R. Panicola, "Withdrawing Nutrition and Hydration," *Health Progress* 82/6 (Nov.-Dec. 2001): 28-33.
13. Daniel P. Sulmasy, "Preserving Life? The Vatican & PVS," *Commonweal* 134/21 (Dec. 7, 2007): 16-18.
14. Bishops of Pennsylvania, "Nutrition and Hydration: Moral Considerations," *Origins* 21/34 (January 30, 1992): 541, 543-53.
15. See, for example, Bishop James McHugh, "Comments After Nancy Cruzan's Death," *Origins* 20/32 (January 17, 1991): 518-19.
16. William E. May et al., "Feeding and Hydrating the Permanently Unconscious and Other Vulnerable Persons," *Issues in Law and Medicine* 3/3 (Winter 1987): 203-11.
17. Texas Catholic Bishops and the Texas Conference of Catholic Health Facilities, "On Withdrawing Artificial Nutrition and Hydration," *Origins* 20/4 (June 7, 1990): 53-55.
18. Committee for Pro-Life Activities of the National Conference of Catholic Bishops, "Nutrition and Hydration: Moral and Pastoral Reflections," *Origins* 21/44 (April 9, 1992): 705-12.
19. Dennis Brodeur, "Is a Decision to Forgo Tube Feeding for Another a Decision to Kill?" *Issues in Law and Medicine* 6/4 (1991): 395-406.
20. David F. Kelly, *Medical Care at the End of Life* (Washington, DC: Georgetown University Press, 2006).
21. President's Commission for the Study of Ethical Problems in Medicine and Biomedical and Behavioral Research, *Deciding to Forego Life-Sustaining Treatment* (March 1983; reprint New York: Concern for Dying).
22. Kevin O'Rourke, OP, "Should Nutrition and Hydration Be Provided to Permanently Unconscious and Other Mentally Disabled Persons?" *Issues in Law and Medicine* 5/2 (1989): 181-96.
23. American Dietetic Association, "Position of The American Dietetic Association: Legal and Ethical Issues in Feeding Permanently Unconscious Patients," *Journal of the American Dietetic Association* 95/2 (February 1995): 231-34.

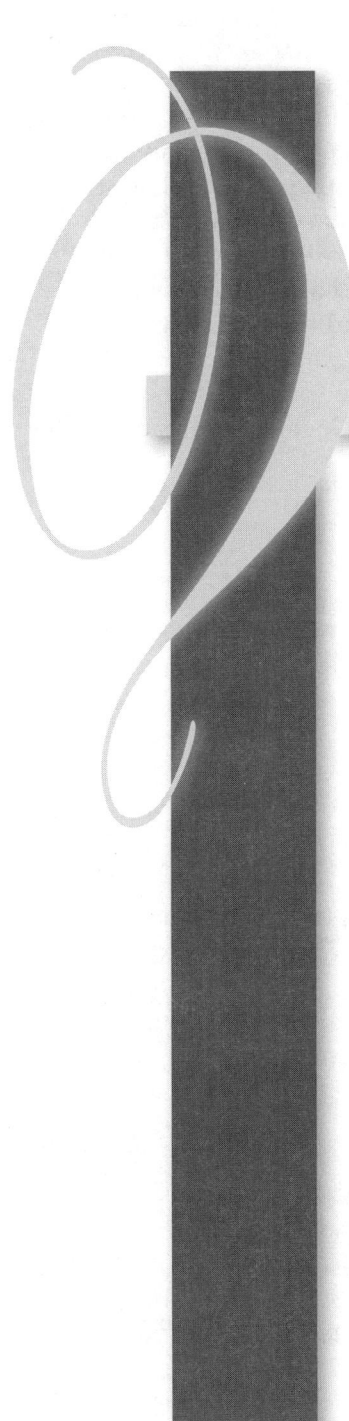

Chapter 10

Euthanasia and Assisted Suicide

Euthanasia and assisted suicide are both deliberate attempts to end a patient's life in order to end his or her suffering. These practices differ in the agent who introduces the immediate and direct cause of death. The act is called *euthanasia* when a person other than the patient directly does something to cause the patient's death. If a doctor injects a patient with an overdose of narcotic medication with the intent of bringing about the patient's death (perhaps in response to the patient's request), this is an act of euthanasia. *Assisted suicide* takes place when someone provides the patient with the means to take his or her own life but the patient is the one who directly initiates the action causing death. If a doctor deliberately prescribes medication so that a patient can take an overdose at home to cause his death, this is a case of assisted suicide. More specifically, this is a case of *physician assisted suicide*. (For the distinction between these practices and forgoing life-sustaining treatments, see chapter 6.)

Euthanasia is considered *voluntary* when it is undertaken at the request of or with the consent of the patient, *involuntary* when it is performed without the patient's consent. If a patient who is physically unable to take his own life asks a doctor to administer an overdose of a narcotic drug, this is an instance of voluntary euthanasia. If a physician administers an overdose of a narcotic drug to an elderly dementia patient solely at the request of the patient's children, this is a case of involuntary euthanasia.

Assisted suicide or euthanasia might be considered when the patient is in the final stages of the dying process, or when the patient has a progressively debilitating disease, or when the patient has a terminal condition or a severely debilitating disease and is in severe pain.

Euthanasia, both voluntary and involuntary, has been practiced in the Netherlands. (1, 2) In the United States, several states have legalized physician assisted suicide. (3, 4)

In this chapter you will learn about:

- arguments presented in favor of euthanasia and assisted suicide;
- objections raised against euthanasia and assisted suicide;
- pain management and other forms of palliative care as an alternative to euthanasia and assisted suicide.

Case Study

Mark Bennett has just finished his training as a physician assistant. Shortly after beginning work at Parkview Memorial Hospital, he encounters a situation he finds very disturbing.

Ruth and Tom Jackson have been married for over forty years. Three years ago, Ruth was found to have stomach and colon cancer. Since that time, she has undergone chemotherapy treatment. However, it was recently discovered that the cancer has spread to Ruth's pancreas.

Ruth has now been hospitalized at Parkview for a week. Her weight is down to 95 pounds, and friends who come to see her remark how much she has "aged." Her pain is constant. Although Ruth is receiving pain medication, it doesn't seem strong enough to really help her.

Tom spent last night at the hospital at his wife's side. Her discomfort was so intense that she kept waking up and wasn't able to sleep well. All Tom could do was sit and hold her hand while she twisted and turned in bed. Several times during the night, Ruth moaned that she wished "it was over."

The next morning Tom asks to talk with PA Mark Bennett. The Jackson and Bennett families have been friends for years, and Tom knew Mark as he was growing up. Tom feels Mark will understand what Ruth is going through.

"I know you can give injections of medications," Tom tells Mark. "I want you to get several doses of Ruth's pain medication, and give it to her all at once to end her suffering. If you don't do this, I will take a pillow and smother Ruth. She's going to die anyway, and I love her too much to allow her to suffer any more."

If something isn't done, Mark fears that Tom will carry out his threat to smother his wife, with dire legal consequences for him. Mark begins to think about what the options are in this case.

* * *

At age 65, Christopher Vaughn decides to sell the jewelry store he started and managed for forty years in a small Midwestern community. The first two years of his retirement are good ones, giving him the opportunity to spend time with his six grandchildren. But then his wife, Roberta, begins to notice behavioral changes in him. After he "got lost" driving home one afternoon, they both agree that he should be checked out medically. It is learned that Christopher is in the very early stages of Alzheimer's disease.

To make matters worse, Roberta dies unexpectedly. Christopher decides to enter Glenview Village, a multi-level facility, in order to "prepare for the future." Initially, Christopher resides in an assisted living apartment, but he understands what is to come as the disease progresses. And, apart from his Alzheimer's disease, his eyesight is beginning to fail and he is starting to have difficulties walking because of arthritis.

Christopher has three children, Monica, Mark, and Amy. Mark and Amy live out of state, so the main care giving responsibilities fall on Christopher's oldest daughter Monica who lives in a nearby city. Monica drives to Glenview Village several times a week to see her father, usually spending half a day with him and taking care of needs around the apartment. Monica never complains, but Christopher worries that she is taking too much time away from her own husband and children in order to care for him. Christopher also worries about the high cost of his present and future care. He knows that people with Alzheimer's disease can still live for a long time, and his retirement "nest egg" really isn't all that much. He doesn't want his children to have to assume the cost of his care, especially with children of their own to educate.

> Christopher dearly loves his six grandchildren, and much prizes the time he has spent with them since his retirement. He wants them to have good memories of their grandfather. He dreads the idea that they will eventually see him in a demented, debilitated state.
>
> During the winter, Christopher suffers a mild stroke which leaves him with some difficulties with swallowing. For this reason, he is seeing Sarah Jones, a speech therapist.
>
> During one therapy session, Christopher asks Sarah if she can help him make contact with Dr. Laura MacDonald. It is rumored around town that Dr. MacDonald has helped two elderly women commit suicide, and Sarah knows this. Sarah is suspicious of Christopher's intent and wonders how she should handle this situation.
>
> ■ ■ ■

The Defense of Euthanasia and Assisted Suicide

What are the arguments that might be offered in support of acts of euthanasia and assisted suicide? How do people try to justify it?

First, these practices are defended as acts of compassion in relieving suffering:

> Many advocates of euthanasia assert that there is a significant number of cases in which even the best medical technology cannot alleviate the physical pain of the terminally ill. Moreover, our technological advances have done little or nothing to help ameliorate the psychological fear and existential anxiety experienced by all at the approach of death, more acutely by some than others. Indeed, the fear of being trapped on life-support machinery is clearly a new and modern fear. These advocates claim that we act out of compassionate concern for our fellow humans when we end their pointless suffering at their own request. (1)

In the first case scenario, Ruth Jackson is in the final stages of the dying process. She is in constant pain, which is not being relieved by medication. She cannot sleep, and wishes for her death. Why not compassionately end her suffering now, as her husband wishes? After all, it is accepted practice to put animals out of their misery. Should we not be at least as kind to human beings?

Another argument offered in favor of euthanasia and assisted suicide is that these practices promote death with dignity. Human dignity "is violated, those who favor assisted suicide/euthanasia maintain, when we are forced to go through an agonizing period of pain and suffering before our lives end." (2) And "our dignity is assaulted, not only by physical pain, but by the depersonalization associated with prolonged use of life-sustaining technology, loss of control over our bodily functions, and the deterioration of our health . . . ". (2) With euthanasia and assisted suicide, a patient can end his life when he is still "himself," and be remembered that way by his loved ones. (5) In the second case scenario, Christopher Vaughn is becoming increasing debilitated physically (arthritis, failing eyesight, stroke). He faces increasing mental deterioration because of Alzheimer's disease. He dreads the idea that his grandchildren will see him in a demented and debilitated state.

Further, a value much emphasized in contemporary health care ethics is patient autonomy (see chapter 1). But "if self-determination is a value, then it is important that each individual be allowed to control the manner, circumstances, and time of death." (1; see also 2) Christopher Vaughn is seeking physician assisted suicide. Although he is in the early stages of Alzheimer's disease, he presumably still has the mental competency to make such a decision, and the principle of autonomy would say that he should have this option.

An analogy with the rightness of decisions to withdraw treatment has also been used to support euthanasia and physician assisted suicide. (2) Consider the following scenario:

> . . . two terminally ill people with the same condition, such as pancreatic cancer, both face a difficult period of dying. Should one suffer respiratory arrest, he could be put on a ventilator, which then could be withdrawn, allowing him to die. Another might not be fortunate enough to arrest. He would continue to live, experiencing pain and suffering until he dies. (2)

It is argued that "there is a lack of equity . . . between the way that these two patients are treated," and that this inequity could be remedied if euthanasia and assisted suicide were made available to the latter. (2) If Ruth Jackson were on a ventilator, removing it might be a way of allowing death to occur and ending her suffering. However, she does not have that option. Neither is Christopher Vaughn currently on any life-prolonging treatments that might be withdrawn to allow his death. Euthanasia and assisted suicide would provide them with the same opportunity for death to occur as have patients who, through "the luck of the draw," are on life-sustaining treatments that can be stopped.

Finally, many believe that there are exceptions to the general prohibition against killing and that taking human life can sometimes be legitimate. Examples might be self-defense, the killing that takes place during a just war and, some would add, capital punishment. Some argue that this list should be expanded to include euthanasia and assisted suicide for the terminally ill and for those suffering from irreversible, progressively debilitating diseases like multiple sclerosis or Alzheimer's. (2) The justification for this expansion is utilitarian (see chapter 1); namely, that the willful taking of life can be morally justified if the good desired outweighs the potential evil and that good cannot be achieved in a less destructive manner. (2) In the case at hand, it is argued that "the greater value could be achieved in a person's life, *taken as a whole*, if he knew that at a certain stage of his dying he would be painlessly put to death rather than be allowed to linger on." (2)

Objections to Euthanasia and Assisted Suicide

A theoretical argument against euthanasia and assisted suicide comes from natural law ethics. Basically, this theory maintains that an action which is in accord with human nature is right while an action which goes against human nature is wrong (see chapter 1). Euthanasia (and assisted suicide) are seen as going against the natural human inclination for self-preservation, and therefore are judged morally wrong:

> Every human being has a natural inclination to continue living. Our reflexes and responses fit us to fight against attackers, flee wild animals, and dodge out of the way of trucks. In our daily lives we exercise the caution and care necessary to protect ourselves. Our bodies are similarly structured for survival right down to the molecular level. When we are cut, our capillaries seal shut, our blood clots, and fibrinogen is produced to start the process of healing the wound. When we are invaded by bacteria, antibodies are produced to fight against the alien organisms, and their remains are swept out of the body by special cells designed for clean-up work. . . .
>
> It is enough, I believe, to recognize that the organization of the human body and our patterns of behavioral responses make the continuation of life a natural goal. By reason alone, then, we can recognize that euthanasia sets us against our own nature. (6)

Arguments of a more pragmatic character are also advanced against euthanasia and assisted suicide. Thus it has been pointed out that medical diagnoses and prognoses can be mistaken. We all know of people who were told they had a short life expectancy because of a disease, and then unexpectedly recovered or substantially outlived the projections for how much time they had left. In particular, states allowing assisted suicide may have a requirement that the patient have six months or less to live in order to be eligible for this procedure. However, data already collected suggest that a significant number of patients live beyond their six-month prognosis. (7) In sum, since medical diagnoses and prognoses are not one hundred percent sure, the concern is that, if euthanasia and assisted suicide are allowed, some people may end their lives needlessly or prematurely. (6)

Further, there is always the possibility of a breakthrough occurring in medical research, making a treatment available that would improve the condition of a patient with a particular disease. Euthanasia and assisted suicide close off this option. (6) For example, Christopher Vaughn is still in the early stages of Alzheimer's disease. Before he experiences severe mental deterioration, treatments might be developed to ameliorate the symptoms of Alzheimer's and allow him more years of a reasonably good quality of life.

Psychological factors can skew a patient's judgment in requesting an end to his life so that the request does not represent his true, rational, underlying desires. Debilitating or life-limiting diseases can cause a patient to become depressed. (7) This may certainly be true in the case of Christopher Vaughn. Even apart from clinical depression, serious illness can distort a patient's judgment:

> Anyone who has been severely ill knows how distorted his judgment became during the worst moments of the illness. Pain and the toxic effect of disease, or the violent reaction to certain surgical procedures may change our capacity for rational and courageous thought. (8)

While it may be true that "some euthanasia candidates will have their lucid moments," yet "how they are to be distinguished from fellow sufferers who do not, or how these instances are to be distinguished from others when the patient is exercising an irrational judgment, is not an easy matter." (8) Moreover, it is not unusual for a patient to undergo mood changes during the course of a day so that he may want euthanasia or assisted suicide "during the morning depression" but "later in the day he will think quite differently, or will have forgotten all about it." (8) The dying can also become socially isolated, so that "we must ask whether the relational bonds of those requesting assisted suicide/euthanasia have been disrupted and whether such requests arise out of despair." (2)

There is also a concern that patients who are difficult or expensive to take care of may feel pressured by other people into opting for euthanasia or assisted suicide when they really do not want this:

Will we not sweep up, in the process, some who are not really tired of life, but think others are tired of them; some who do not really want to die, but who feel they should not live on, because to do so when there looms the legal alternative of euthanasia is to do a selfish or cowardly act? Will not some feel an obligation to have themselves "eliminated" in order that funds allocated for their terminal care might be better used by their families or, financial worries aside, in order to relieve their families of the emotional strain involved? (8)

For example, Christopher Vaughn's oldest daughter Monica drives from a nearby city several times a week to see him, usually spending half a day with him and taking care of needs around the apartment. Christopher worries that she is taking too much time away from her own husband and children in order to care for him. He also worries about the high cost of his present and future care since he knows that people with Alzheimer's disease can live for a long time. His retirement "nest egg" really isn't all that much, and he doesn't want his children to have to assume the cost of his care, especially with children of their own to educate. Altogether, these are subtle pressures that may be pushing Christopher to consider assisted suicide.

Further, there is fear that a slippery slope effect will occur. In other words, there is fear that if we allow euthanasia and assisted suicide in some cases, the practice might expand to include other cases in which these practices are highly questionable. For example, we might start out with voluntary euthanasia and assisted suicide, wherein life is ended at the request of the patient. But this might expand to cases of involuntary euthanasia in which someone other than the patient decides that a patient's life is to be ended:

> . . . if the warrant for assisted suicide/euthanasia is to relieve suffering, there is no reason why these practices should be limited to those who are competent. Why not provide killing for those who are suffering and can no longer speak for themselves? If suffering provides a moral warrant for voluntary euthanasia, it should also provide a warrant for nonvoluntary euthanasia. (2)

Indeed, "the experience of the Netherlands shows that nonvoluntary euthanasia can follow voluntary euthanasia, even when this is not planned." (2) Or, we might start out with allowing euthanasia and assisted suicide for those who are terminally ill and find it expanding to the chronically ill and incurable, and even to those with psychiatric disorders. (2) In the case of Dr. Jack Kevorkian, a Michigan physician who openly practiced assisted suicide, the practice extended to a person whose condition was not life-threatening and may well have been treatable. The thirty-fifth person he helped commit suicide was Judith Curren, a woman suffering from chronic fatigue syndrome, a weight problem, and depression. (9)

Finally, the impact of euthanasia and assisted suicide on health care providers and services should be considered. Fundamentally, persons in the health care professions are healers. It is feared that combining killing with healing would result in confusion and distrust of health care providers among patients, and undermine the relationship of health care providers with their patients. (2) Further, in the era of managed care and cost containment, euthanasia and assisted suicide could come to "be seen as cheaper alternatives for health care systems than palliative care for the dying or ameliorative treatment for the incurable." (2) Indeed, "in a social context where medical care is already limited according to race, gender, and ability to pay, a policy of euthanasia might be implemented more readily for the poor, racial minorities, and women than for others." (2)

Managing Pain and Relieving Suffering

The societal movement towards euthanasia and assisted suicide did not arise in a vacuum. Opponents of these practices see this movement as resulting from a failure to provide good care for the dying:

> Many who care for the dying tell us that people are generally not afraid to die. They fear, rather, the process of dying, especially the dependency, helplessness, and pain that so often accompany terminal illness. . . .
>
> One of the major arguments of euthanasia advocates is that for some people dying is too painful to endure and so bringing about death by lethal injection or assisted suicide is the only merciful way to end the pain and suffering. (9)

Thus, some opponents of euthanasia and assisted suicide are campaigning for better palliative care for the dying. (11) Recognizing that a cure cannot be achieved, this is medical care aimed at relieving pain and other distressing symptoms of the dying process. As one proponent of palliative care states, ". . . people involved in health care have now what may be a brief window of opportunity to increase their efforts to improve and refine palliative medicine and hospice practice so that fewer and fewer persons imagine that PAD [physician-assisted dying] is their only hope, as they live in fear of unrelieved suffering and indignity in their dying as a consequence of medical neglect." (11)

Various factors can be barriers to good pain management. One factor is a lack of training of health care workers in good pain management techniques. Some health care workers do not know what is available for pain management and how to use it effectively. (12) This may be true in the case of Ruth Jackson. Due to her cancer, Ruth is described as suffering intense pain, but "studies indicate that as many as 95 percent" of cancer patients "*can* get good pain relief if skilled practitioners administer the right medications in the right ways." (12)

Another factor that can negatively impact good pain management is fear of the patient becoming addicted to the pain medication. (13, 14) However, a distinction can be made between *addiction* and *drug dependence*. In the case of drug dependency, the drug has a medical value for the person taking it. The dependency is a physical, rather than a psychological, problem. Withdrawal symptoms will occur if the drug is taken away suddenly, so that the drug needs to be taken away gradually, over a period of time. Addiction, on the other hand, is a psychological problem. The drug has no medical value for the person taking it, but the individual desires it and is driven to obtain it. (14, 15)

If Ruth Jackson had been given pain medication in doses sufficient to control her severe pain, she would undoubtedly have become physically dependent on it, but this does not mean that she should be considered an addict. Moreover, in the case of someone who is dying, like Ruth Jackson, the pain medication need never be stopped to cause withdrawal symptoms. (15) Other cultural factors may also hinder good pain management. In the minds of some people the term "narcotic" (that is, opioid) automatically evokes an image of street drugs. (14) Unfortunately, the stigma attached to opioids may carry over into the health care setting, where such drugs have perfectly legitimate uses. (16)

From an ethical point of view, the classic question about pain management at the end of life has concerned the use of medications that may hasten death. Specifically, there has been concern about narcotics depressing respiration and, in this way, having a secondary effect of hastening the patient's death. Such a secondary effect has made some health care providers hesitant about administering these pain medications for fear that they are engaging in an act of euthanasia. (15, 17) These concerns might well arise in a case like that of Ruth Jackson, where high doses of opioids would likely be needed to control her severe cancer pain.

Traditionally, the answer has been that it is ethically permissible to use medications to relieve pain that may have a side effect of hastening the time of death based on the *principle of double effect*. (12, 13) This ethical principle applies to situations in which a single action will have two different consequences. One of the consequences is perfectly good and is what is intended. The second consequence, however, is bad and is not really wanted, but it comes along as a side effect of the action. The principle of double effect says that it is ethically permissible to take an action with such double consequences. More exactly, the principle of double effect can be stated as follows:

> This doctrine, which is designed to provide moral guidance for an action that could have at least one bad and one good effect, holds that such an action is permissible if it satisfies these four conditions: (1) The act itself must be morally good or neutral (for example, administering a pain-killer); (2) only the good consequences of the action must be intended (relief of the patient's suffering); (3) the good effect must not be produced by means of the evil effect (the relief of suffering must not be produced by the patient's death); (4) there must be some weighty reason for permitting the evil (the relief of great suffering, which can only be achieved through a high risk of death). (17)

Intent is critical in using the principle of double effect. It must be pain relief, not the patient's death, that is intended in administering the medication. But how does one know someone's intent in administering pain medication? This is one way: if a patient's pain is relieved by a certain dosage level of the pain medication, the level will not be deliberately increased to risk depression of respiration (and death). This indicates that the intent is indeed to relieve pain.

Fortunately, this ethical concern about pain medication is becoming outdated. First of all, "there is some evidence that administering narcotic agents in amounts sufficient to provide adequate pain relief may extend, rather than shorten, life." (15) This is so because "patients without pain are more likely to accept a greater degree of nourishment, to be more active and less depressed, and to be more open to other treatment possibilities," and, "as a result, they may live longer." (15) Second, more is now known about how to administer pain medication in a way that avoids depression of respiration:

> Health care professionals who are accustomed to giving one to two milligrams of morphine in the emergency room or coronary care unit for the relief of moderate acute pain need to know that some patients may need, and can tolerate, 1,000 milligrams or more of morphine per hour, as in intravenous infusion, to control the ferocious pain of some cancers. Such doses are not reached overnight but infusions are judiciously titrated upwards in measured increments until pain is contained. In this way respiratory distress does not occur, since unrelieved pain acts as a physiological antagonist to the respiratory depressant effect of the opiate drug. (10)

Finally, it is now recognized that respiratory depression and arrest is a normal part of the dying process, and we need to be careful not to falsely see it as caused by pain medication:

> However, current medical research raises questions about the need to apply the principle of double effect to pain management. As the chair of the Wisconsin Cancer Pain Initiative stated in correspondence to the Council of Ethical and Judicial Affairs of the American Medical Association, "Death from respiratory depression is exceedingly rare in patients with cancer who chronically receive opioid analgesics for pain. As a person nears death, there is deterioration in respiratory function. However, these respiratory changes should not be confused with the effects of opioids. (13)

In sum, there is no reason to withhold adequate doses of pain medication from dying patients for fear of hastening their deaths.

On some occasions the administration of medication adequate to relieve severe pain may impair a patient's mental functioning, causing confusion, reducing decision-making capacity, or even reducing or suppressing consciousness. In respect for patient autonomy, the patient should be consulted when pain medication is likely to have these effects. The patient should have the opportunity to decide what level of pain, if any, she is prepared to tolerate as a trade-off for mental clarity. (15) The patient may want to remain mentally alert for some period in order to take care of unfinished business matters, visit with family members and friends, or prepare spiritually for death.

While most pain can be relieved, there is a residue of unrelievable pain. It has been estimated that "between 5% and 35% of hospice patients have intractable symptoms in the last week of life" which may include "pain, shortness of breath, dyspnea, nausea and vomiting." (18) In these cases, some find euthanasia or assisted suicide attractive as ways of relieving the suffering of patients who are already dying. (19) An alternative in these cases is sedation to the point of unconsciousness on a continuing basis:

> If the only troubling issue that arises . . . is that of having to accept unconsciousness in order to avoid severe pain, this is a morally acceptable course. . . . It may be that a brief life of nearly continuous sedation is not of great merit, even though it is better than any other life that can be made available. . . . However, continuous sedation achieves a humane and compassionate period of dying for patient, caregivers, and family without precipitating the very serious concerns about "slippery slopes"

that arise with acceptance of direct killing. Therefore, sedation is the best policy in the unusual instance of pain so severe that it cannot be relieved while still keeping the patient awake. (20)

This practice is referred to as *terminal sedation* or *palliative sedation*. (21) This course of action might be an option of last resort in the case of Ruth Jackson.

While we have been focusing on the management of physical pain, it is important to keep in mind that the suffering that accompanies the dying process goes beyond physical pain. Providing emotional and psychological support for those who are ill is likewise advocated as part of good care of the dying. As stated in one document opposing euthanasia:

> The pleas of gravely ill people who sometimes ask for death are not to be understood as implying a true desire for euthanasia; in fact it is almost always a case of an anguished plea for help and love. What a sick person needs, besides medical care, is love, the human and supernatural warmth with which the sick person can and ought to be surrounded by all those close to him or her, parents and children, doctors and nurses. (22)
>
> As for those who work in the medical profession, they ought to neglect no means of making all their skill available to the sick and the dying; but they should also remember how much more necessary it is to provide them with the comfort of boundless kindness and heartfelt charity. (22)

Advancing the cause of palliative care is one area in which proponents and opponents of euthanasia and assisted suicide may find some common ground. For even some who believe euthanasia and assisted suicide are morally permissible in some cases still advocate trying palliative care as the first course of action:

> The new Quill plan proposes to use palliative care experts to review *all* requests for assisted suicide or euthanasia. The specialist in comfort care would talk with the patient and primary physician, and review the medical records and treatments that have already been used. . . . if the palliative care doctor finds that the patient's request for euthanasia comes from inadequate treatment of his symptoms, wrote Quill and his colleagues, "The process of consultation might lead to improved pain management or the use of other means of comfort care." In any case, a patient who had not yet received adequate comfort care would be offered better treatment of symptoms, not death. (19)

CHAPTER SUMMARY

Key Terms and Concepts

euthanasia: a person other than the patient intentionally performs an action that is the direct, immediate cause of the patient's death.
voluntary euthanasia: an act of euthanasia undertaken at the request of the patient.
involuntary euthanasia: an act of euthanasia undertaken without the consent of the patient.
assisted suicide: another person provides a patient with the means to take his or her own life.
principle of double effect: It is ethically permissible to take a course of action that has an evil effect accompanying a good one provided that the act itself is ethically good or neutral, only the good consequence of the action is intended, the good effect is not produced by means of the evil effect, and there is some weighty reason for permitting the evil.

Key Points

- Arguments given *in support of* euthanasia and assisted suicide include the following:

  * Euthanasia and assisted suicide are acts of compassion in relieving suffering.
  * Euthanasia and assisted suicide promote death with dignity.
  * Choosing the time of one's death is an exercise of autonomy.
  * Euthanasia and assisted suicide provide the same opportunity for death that is available to patients able to have life-sustaining treatments withdrawn.
  * We already recognize some cases in which it is legitimate to take human life, and euthanasia and assisted suicide should be included.

- Arguments *against* euthanasia and assisted suicide include the following:

  * These practices violate natural law in going against the natural human inclination for self-preservation.
  * If euthanasia and assisted suicide are allowed, some patients may end their lives needlessly or prematurely because medical diagnoses and prognoses can be mistaken.

* There is always the possibility of a breakthrough occurring in medical research that would make a treatment available to improve the condition of a patient with a particular disease.
* Psychological factors (e.g., depression, mood swings, distortion of judgment caused by illness, feelings of social isolation) can skew a patient's judgment in requesting an end to his life so that the request does not represent his true, rational, underlying desires.
* Patients could feel pressured to end their lives by financial considerations or in order to relieve significant others of the strains of care giving.
* Allowing euthanasia and assisted suicide in the case of terminally ill patients by their request or with their consent could have a slippery slope effect, leading to involuntary euthanasia and even to ending the lives of patients whose conditions are not life-threatening and may be treatable.
* Euthanasia and assisted suicide are incompatible with the traditional role of health care workers as healers, and could lead to a decline in the quality of medical care made available to debilitated and dying patients.

- Good pain management and palliative care may remove a motive for engaging in euthanasia or assisted suicide. Care should address the emotional and psychological, as well as the physical, needs of a patient.
- According to the principle of double effect, it is ethically permissible to use sufficient medication to control pain although that medication has a side effect of hastening a patient's death. However, this side effect of pain medication may be avoidable and not as prevalent as once thought.
- In the case of severe pain that cannot otherwise be relieved, terminal/palliative sedation (sedating a patient to the point of unconsciousness) may be an alternative to euthanasia or assisted suicide.
- Both proponents and opponents of euthanasia and assisted suicide see the need for providing better palliative care for the dying.

FOR FURTHER DISCUSSION

1. Critically assess the arguments offered *in favor* of euthanasia and assisted suicide. Do these arguments hold up? Can any replies be made to them? Are some of the arguments good ones while others are not plausible? Do the same for the arguments put forward *against* euthanasia and assisted suicide.
2. Consider the case of Ruth Jackson at the beginning of the chapter. After critically assessing the arguments on both sides and considering the facts of

the case, do you think that euthanasia would be an ethically correct course of action in the case of Ruth?
3. Consider the case of Christopher Vaughn at the beginning of the chapter. After critically assessing the arguments on both sides and the facts of the case, do you think that physician assisted suicide would be an ethically correct course of action for Christopher?
4. In our first case scenario, Tom Jackson asks physician assistant Mark Bennett to euthanize his wife. Suppose you were Mark Bennett. How do you think you would react to this situation? What would you say to Tom? What courses of action might be options for handling this situation?
5. In our second case scenario, Christopher Vaughn essentially asks speech therapist Sarah Jones to help him arrange an assisted suicide. Suppose you were Sarah Jones. How do you think you would react to this situation? What would you say to Christopher? What courses of action might be options for handling this situation?
6. If you are a member of a church, research your denomination's views on euthanasia and assisted suicide. Then compare in class the positions and statements of various denominations. (Keep in mind that you may be caring for patients whose decisions on death and dying issues will be guided by the position of their religious denomination.)
7. In 1997 the United States Supreme Court rendered a judgment in two cases concerning assisted suicide, *Washington v. Glucksberg* and *Vacco v. Quill*. The Supreme Court put the question of the legal permissibility of assisted suicide in the hands of the states, leaving it to individual states to decide whether to allow and experiment with assisted suicide. (11) Have a debate about whether assisted suicide should be made legal in your state.

References

1. Michael Manning, *Euthanasia and Physician-Assisted Suicide Killing or Caring?* (New York/Mahwah, NJ: 1998).
2. Committee on Medical Ethics of the Episcopal Diocese of Washington, DC, *Assisted Suicide and Euthanasia Christian Moral Perspectives* (Harrisburg, PA: Morehouse Publishing, 1997).
3. State of Oregon, "Physician Assisted Suicide," http://egov.oregon.gov/DHS/ph/pas/ index.shtml. Accessed January 2009.

4. Kevin B. O'Reilly, "Washington becomes 2nd state to allow physician-assisted suicide," amednews.com (November 24, 2008), http://www.ama-assn.org/amednews/2008/11/24/ prsb1124.htm. Accessed January 2009.
5. *Help Me Die.* Fanlight Productions, videocassette.
6. J. Gay-Williams, "The Wrongfulness of Euthanasia" in Ronald Munson (ed.), *Intervention and Reflection: Basic Issues in Medical Ethics,* 8th ed. (Belmont, CA: Thomson Wadsworth, 2008).
7. Herbert Hendin and Kathleen Foley, "Physician-Assisted Suicide in Oregon: A Medical Perspective," *Michigan Law Review* 106 (June 2008): 1613-39, http://www.spiorg.org/publications/HendinFoley_MichiganLawReview.pdf. Accessed January 2009.
8. Yale Kamisar, "From Euthanasia Legislation: Some Non-Religious Objections" in A.B. Downing (ed.), *Euthanasia and the Right to Die* (New York: Humanities Press, 1970).
9. Chicago Tribune, "Kevorkian Steps Over a Fine Line," reprinted in the (Dubuque) *Telegraph-Herald,* August 23, 1996.
10. Catholic Health Association of the United States, *Care of the Dying* (St. Louis: Catholic Health Association of the United States, 1993).
11. James F. Bresnahan, "Palliative Care or Assisted Suicide?" *America* (March 14, 1998): 16-21.
12. Phebe Saunders Haugen, "Pain Relief: Legal Aspects of Pain Relief for the Dying," *Minnesota Medicine* 80 (November 1997): 15-18.
13. Thomas E. Elliott, "Pain Control at the End of Life," *Minnesota Medicine* 80 (November 1997): 27-32.
14. *Quality of Mercy: A Case for Better Pain Management,* prod. Richard J. Adler, Filmmakers Library, videocassette.
15. Hastings Center, *Guidelines on the Termination of Life-Sustaining Treatment and the Care of the Dying* (Briarcliff Manor, NY: Hastings Center, 1987).
16. Russell K. Portenoy et al., "Pain Management and Chemical Dependency," *Journal of the American Medical Association* 278/7 (August 20, 1997): 592-3.
17. President's Commission for the Study of Ethical Problems in Medicine and Biomedical and Behavioral Research, *Deciding to Forego Life-Sustaining Treatment* (1983; reprint New York: Concern for Dying).
18. Kevin B. O'Reilly, "AMA Meeting: AMA OKs palliative sedation for terminally ill," amednews.com (July 7, 2008), http://www.ama-assn.org/amednews/2008/07/07/prsi0707. Accessed January 2009.
19. Lonny Shavelson, *A Chosen Death: The Dying Confront Assisted Suicide* (New York: Simon & Schuster, 1995).

20. Joanne Lynn, "Morpheus or Death: The Case of Nicholas Miklovick" in Cynthia B. Cohen (ed.), *Casebook on the Termination of Life-Sustaining Treatment and the Care of the Dying* (Bloomington, IN: Indiana University Press, 1988).
21. David F. Kelly, *Medical Care at the End of Life* (Washington, DC: Georgetown University Press, 2006).
22. Vatican Congregation for the Doctrine of the Faith, *Declaration on Euthanasia* (Washington, DC: United States Catholic Conference, 1980).

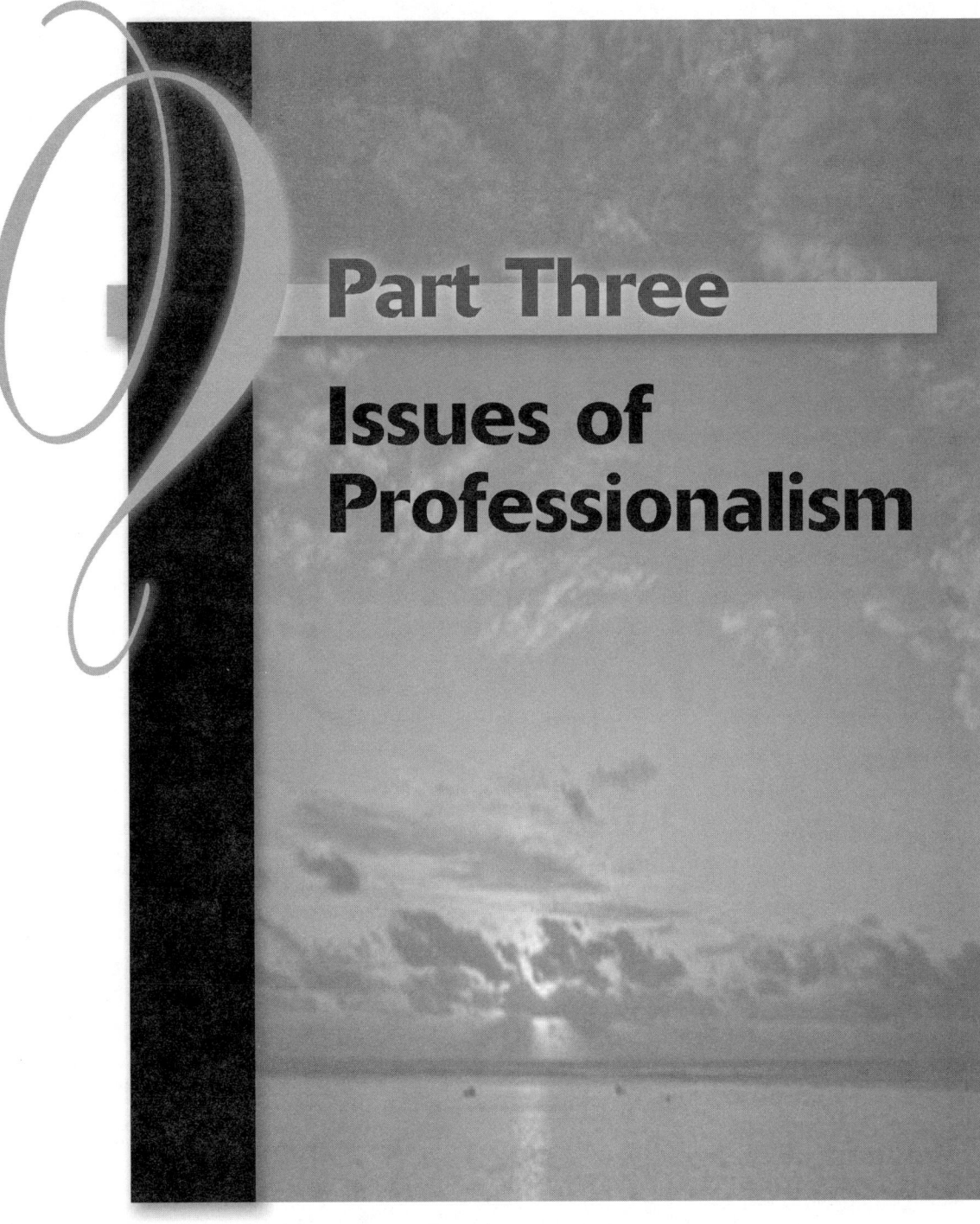

Part Three

Issues of Professionalism

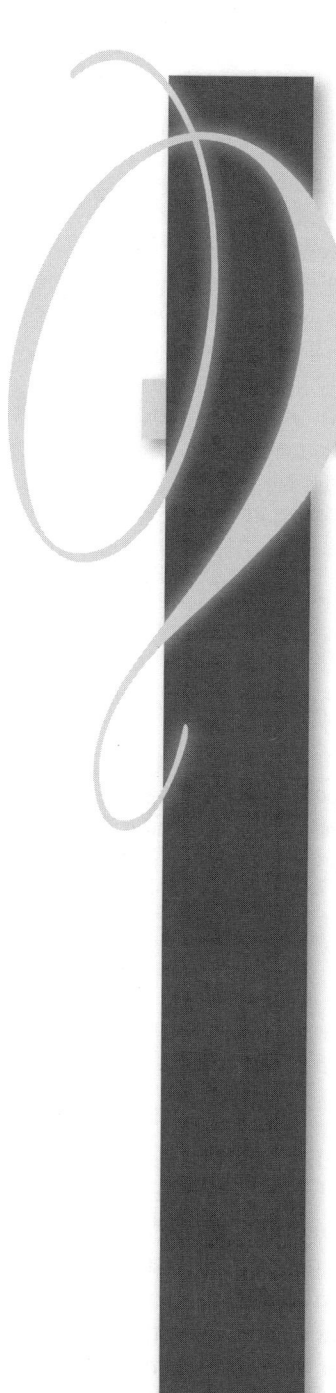

Chapter 11

Confidentiality

Leaks of supposedly confidential or privileged information to the media have become commonplace in American society. Such leaks are a way of life. This attitude makes it harder to appreciate why confidentiality is emphasized and expected in health care. Yet confidentiality goes back to the Hippocratic oath: "Whatever I see or hear, professionally or privately, which ought not be divulged, I will keep secret and tell no one." (1)

In this chapter you will learn about:

- the reasons why confidentiality is an important value in health care;
- the ethical principle governing confidentiality;
- when it is ethically legitimate to break confidentiality;
- current challenges to maintaining confidentiality;
- governmental regulations pertaining to confidentiality in health care.

Case Study

Eleanor Murray works in the medical records department at Lakeland Hospital. One day her supervisor asks her to review some medical records to check on insurance claims for a particular company. One of the files she is supposed to review belongs to Roger Faber. In looking through the file, Eleanor notices that Roger has undergone testing for the gene for Huntington's disease because of a history of this disease in his family, and has tested positive. Huntington's disease affects persons during their adult years, and involves worsening gait, constant uncontrollable movement, and personality changes. Death usually comes ten to fifteen years after the onset of symptoms. If someone has the gene for Huntington's disease, it is almost inevitable that he will eventually be affected by the disease.

This discovery upsets Eleanor very much since her sister Jean is engaged to marry Roger. Does her sister know about Roger's genetic status? How will this affect their marriage? Should Jean be burdened with heavy caregiving responsibilities for Roger? Will Jean have to forgo having her own biological children to prevent Huntington's disease from being passed on to them?

Eleanor has always been protective of her sister Jean. Eleanor knows that any information she sees in medical records is supposed to be kept confidential. At the same time, she doesn't want to see her sister get hurt. She struggles with the question of whether she should break confidentiality and tell Jean about Roger's genetic status.

■ ■ ■

Why Confidentiality Is a Value in Health Care

There are several justifications for maintaining confidentiality in health care practice. Based on the ethical principle of autonomy (see chapter 1), an individual has a right to control personal information and to protect privacy. (2) A health care professional would not "show proper respect for the patient's autonomy and privacy if he or she does not uphold the confidentiality of the professional-patient relationship." (3) Consequentialist ethics (see chapter 1) also provides an underpinning for confidentiality. (3, 4) For "if patients could not trust physicians to conceal some information from third parties, patients would be reluctant to disclose full and forthright information or to authorize a complete examination and a full battery of tests." (4) And, "without such information, physicians would not be able to make accurate diagnoses and prognoses or to recommend the best course of treatment." (4) The concern that, without assurance of confidentiality, patients may not disclose all relevant information to health care providers or be deterred from seeking treatment altogether is reinforced by the fact that some medical problems are quite personal, such as infertility and sexually transmitted diseases. It is also reinforced by the fact that some diseases, such as AIDS and mental illness, carry a social stigma and may lead to discrimination. (2, 5)

To appreciate the value of confidentiality, just consider what appears on the evening news when the President of the United States or another prominent person has a serious health problem and must have surgery or other treatment. Would you want this kind of information broadcast about yourself?

The Principle of Confidentiality

As an ethical principle, *there is a strong prima facie obligation to maintain confidentiality about medical information.* (4) In others words, there is an expectation that confidentiality be maintained about medical information, unless the value of maintaining confidentiality is overridden by exceptional circumstances. The exceptional circumstances which are recognized to justify breaking confidentiality are *substantial threats to others, to the public interest, or to the patient.* (4)

The ethical theories that support maintaining confidentiality also allow for exceptions to the rule. The ethical theory of principalism (see chapter 1) recognizes the principle of nonmaleficence (the duty to avoid harm) as well as the principle of autonomy, with nonmaleficence sometimes limiting and taking precedence over autonomy. (2) Consequentialist ethics (see chapter 1) requires that "we compare the benefits of keeping confidences with the benefits of revealing confidential information in circumstances in which the information is desperately needed by another party." (3) And "if through this comparison it turns out that there is an overriding duty to warn persons who might be seriously harmed if confidentiality were maintained, then confidentiality is not an absolute duty." (3)

In some cases breaking confidentiality may be considered ethically *permissible.* In other cases, an argument might be made that it is morally *obligatory* to do so; for example, when there is a high probability of major harm coming to a person other than the patient. (4)

What are examples of cases in which breaking confidentiality would be considered legitimate from an ethical point of view? One example involves the transmission of HIV/AIDS to another person, and hence, the transmission of a potentially fatal disease:

> In one case, after several weeks of dry persistent coughing and night sweats, a bi-sexual man visited his family physician, who arranged for a test to determine whether he had antibodies to HIV. The physician informed the patient of a positive test, of the risk of infection for his wife, and of the risk that their children might lose both parents. The patient refused to tell his wife and insisted that the physician maintain absolute confidentiality. The physician reluctantly yielded to this demand. Only in the last few weeks of his life did the patient allow the physician to inform his wife of the nature of the husband's illness, and a test then showed that she too was antibody-positive for HIV. When symptoms appeared a year later, she angrily, and we think appropriately, accused the physician of violating his moral responsibilities to her and to her children. This case presents a high probability (if we assume unprotected sexual intercourse) of a major harm to an identifiable individual—the paradigm case of a justified breach of confidentiality. (4)

Or again, breaking confidentiality may be necessary in the case of involuntary commitment proceedings for a patient who is apt to commit suicide or engage in self-mutilating behavior. This breach of confidentiality falls into the category of preventing serious harm to the patient himself. Legally, health care workers may be required to report cases of child abuse, gunshot wounds, and cases of contagious diseases. (4)

However, it should be emphasized that such breaches of confidentiality are *exceptional cases*. Apart from legally mandated reporting requirements, health care workers should be extremely cautious about breaking confidentiality. It should always be a "last resort," after alternative courses of action have been explored and failed. (4)

Special Challenges to Maintaining Confidentiality

Living in a small community "where everybody knows everybody else" poses a special challenge to maintaining confidentiality about health information. A patient may find a member of her church or a neighbor, or even a cousin or relative by marriage, among the staff working at the local medical clinic where she seeks care. However, challenges for maintaining confidentiality are not limited to this kind of setting. In general, concern is being voiced about the erosion of the confidential status of medical information.

One challenge to be met is the large number of health care workers involved in the care of a particular patient who can (and need to) have access to his medical records:

> A patient of mine with mild chronic obstructive pulmonary disease was transferred from the surgical intensive-care unit to a surgical nursing floor two days after an elective cholecystectomy. On the day of the transfer, the patient saw a respiratory therapist writing in his medical chart (the therapist was recording the results of an arterial blood gas analysis) and became concerned about the confidentiality of his hospital records. The patient threatened to leave the hospital prematurely unless I could guarantee that the confidentiality of his hospital record would be respected.
>
> The patient's complaint prompted me to enumerate the number of persons who had both access to his hospital record and a reason to examine it. I was amazed to learn that at least 25 and possibly as many as 100 health professionals and administrative personnel at our university hospital had access to the patient's record and that all of them had a legitimate need, indeed a professional responsibility, to open and use that chart. These persons included 6 attending physicians (the primary physician, the surgeon, the pulmonary consultant, and others); 12 house officers (medical, surgical, intensive-care unit, and "covering" house staff); 20 nursing personnel (on three shifts); 6 respiratory therapists; 3 nutritionists; 2 clinical pharmacists; 15 students (from medicine, nursing, respiratory therapy, and clinical pharmacy); 4 unit secretaries; 4 hospital financial officers; and 4 chart reviewers (utilization review, quality assurance review, tissue review, and insurance auditor). It is of interest that this patient's problem was straightforward, and he therefore did not require many other technical and support services that the modern hospital provides.
>
> ... I suggested to the patient that these people were all involved in providing or supporting his health-care services. They were, I assured him, working for him. Despite my reassurances the patient was obviously distressed and retorted, "I always believed that medical confidentiality was part of a doctor's code of ethics. Perhaps you should tell me just what you people mean by 'confidentiality'!" (6)

One way of responding to this problem is for health care facilities and services to emphasize confidentiality as a job expectation of everyone involved in patient care, whether directly or indirectly, and no matter what his or her particular job is. In fact, it has been suggested that job descriptions for health care workers should explicitly mention respect for confidentiality among job qualifications, that all employees who have access to patient information should be asked to sign a confidentiality agreement annually, and that one standard by which a health care worker's job performance should be evaluated is his demonstrated respect for patient confidentiality. (7)

HIPAA Regulations

In 1996 the United States Congress enacted the Health Insurance Portability and Accountability Act (HIPAA). In addition to requirements concerning the transferability of health insurance, this legislation provides a comprehensive framework for regulating the standardization, security, and privacy of health information. The HIPAA statute as such focuses on the electronic exchange of health information. However, as implemented by the U.S. Department of Health and Human Services, HIPAA regulations are much broader and govern essentially all collection, maintenance, transmission, use, and disclosure of "individually identifiable health information." The regulations address standards for transactions (such as health claims and health care payments) to enable the electronic interchange of health information, for a unique health identifier for each individual, for code sets for appropriate data elements for transactions, for security of health information, for electronic signatures, for transfer of information among health plans, and for privacy. (8) The privacy standards in particular interface with the ethical issue of confidentiality.

The Privacy Rule mandates that health care facilities and services have in place privacy policies and procedures appropriate for their services, notify patients about their privacy rights and how their information can be used or disclosed, train employees in understanding the privacy practices, appoint a privacy official responsible for seeing that the privacy policies and procedures are implemented, and safeguard patients' records. (9)

Because allied health professionals handle patient medical records and requests for information from these records, they need to be informed about HIPAA regulations regarding what information can be released about patients' conditions and treatments. (9) Basically, HIPAA allows the use and disclosure of individually identifiable health information for purposes of treatment, payment, and health care operations; all other cases of use or disclosure of such information require a specific authorization by the patient. (9)

To be compliant with HIPAA, a host of daily practices and procedures within a health care facility must be addressed. Do health care workers ever discuss patients among themselves or with family members in public areas of the facility? Do phone conversations occur in an area where patient information can be overheard? Are computer monitors positioned in such a way that unauthorized persons can see information about patients? Are fax machines monitored to ensure that material with patient information is not left available to unauthorized personnel? Are documents with patient information turned face down to avoid observation by visitors? (9) At first glance, such concerns may seem unwarrantedly detailed, onerous, and just another example of governmental bureaucracy. From a more positive perspective, they can be viewed as raising our consciousness about the many arenas in which the concept of confidentiality has applicability.

CHAPTER SUMMARY

Key Terms and Concepts

principle of confidentiality: a strong prima facie obligation exists to maintain confidentiality about medical information. This obligation can be overridden by substantial threats to others, to the public interest, or to the patient.

HIPAA (Health Insurance Portability and Accountability Act): federal legislation that includes mandatory protections for individually identifiable health information.

Key Points

- Confidentiality is important in health care because, if it is not maintained, patients may be deterred from seeking treatment they need or may not want to disclose all the information necessary for effective treatment.
- Ethically, there is an expectation that health care professionals maintain confidentiality about medical information to which they have access. The cases in which breaking confidentiality may be judged ethically permissible or even obligatory are the exception rather than the rule.
- A challenge to maintaining confidentiality in today's health care climate is the large number of health care workers involved in the care of a particular patient.
- Governmental regulations established by HIPAA have reinforced confidentiality in health care and spelled out concretely how it should be put into practice.

FOR FURTHER DISCUSSION

1. Consider the case of Eleanor Murray at the beginning of this chapter. Through her work in the medical records department of a hospital she has learned that Roger Faber, the fiancé of her sister Jean, has tested positive for Huntington's disease. She is debating whether she should break confidentiality and convey this information to her sister.

   - *Eleanor has to weigh the pros and cons of breaking confidentiality in this situation. What are the pros? The cons?*
   - *Role play a conversation between Eleanor and Jean in which Eleanor has decided to break confidentiality and to tell Jean about Roger's genetic status. What might be Jean's reaction if this information is news to her? On the other hand, what might be Jean's reaction if she already knows about Roger's genetic status?*
   - *Considering the ethical principle governing confidentiality, is it justifiable for Eleanor to break confidentiality? Are there any relevant differences between this situation and the case of HIV/AIDS presented in the chapter as a "paradigm case of a justified breach of confidentiality"?*
   - *Considering HIPAA regulations, is it legally permissible for Eleanor to break confidentiality?*
   - *Eleanor is genuinely concerned about the future welfare of her sister. Is there any way Eleanor can handle this situation without breaking confidentiality about the medical record she has seen?*

2. St. Margaret's Hospital is located in a small, rural community. The population of the town is 5,000, and it is surrounded by farms. It is a community that prides itself on being "neighborly."

   Jerry Johnson is a physical therapist at St. Margaret's. While he is shopping in the grocery store one evening, an elderly neighbor, Mrs. Todd, stops to talk with him. Mrs. Todd knows that a little boy down the street from her was hospitalized yesterday after being hit by a car. She asks Jerry if he knows how this little boy is doing.

   Jerry has been giving treatments to the little boy since he arrived at the hospital. Without thinking, Jerry gives Mrs. Todd a fairly detailed report on the boy's injuries and the progress he is making towards recovery. After all, she seems as concerned about him as if he were her own grandchild!

Jerry broke confidentiality by sharing medical information about the injured boy with his neighbor. Clearly, this breach was neither ethically justified nor legally permissible. It is all too easy for health care workers to break confidentiality in casual conversations without thinking. What kind of responses might health care workers prepare to have ready in these kinds of situations?

3. At Oaklawn Community Hospital all the physical therapy equipment is located in one large room. Several patients and their therapists are usually present in the room at the same time. Sometimes family members stay with the patients during the therapy sessions. In this kind of setting, what can be done to maintain confidentiality for individual patients?

References

1. "Confidentiality" in Ronald Munson (ed.), *Intervention and Reflection: Basic Issues in Medical Ethics*, 8th ed. (Belmont, CA: Thomson Wadsworth, 2008).
2. Morton E. Winston, "AIDS, Confidentiality, and The Right to Know," *Public Affairs Quarterly* 2/2 (April 1988): 91-104.
3. Tom L. Beauchamp and LeRoy Walters (eds.), *Contemporary Issues in Bioethics*, 6th ed. (Belmont, CA: Thomson Wadsworth, 2003).
4. Tom L. Beauchamp & James F. Childress, *Principles of Biomedical Ethics*, 5th ed. (New York: Oxford, 2001).
5. California Supreme Court, *Tarasoff v. Regents of the University of California*, 131 *California Reporter* 14 (July 1, 1976).
6. Mark Siegler, "Confidentiality in Medicine—A Decrepit Concept," *New England Journal of Medicine* 307/24 (9 December 1982): 518-21.
7. Ida Critelli Schick, "Protecting Patients' Privacy," *Health Progress* (May-June 1998): 26-31.
8. Maureen Weaver, Jeanette C. Schreiber, Michelle Wilcox DeBarge, Catherine P. Baatz, Wiggin & Dana, LLP, *The HIPAA Handbook for Implementing the Federal Privacy Rule in the Long-Term Care Setting* (Washington, DC: American Association of Homes and Services for the Aging, 2001).
9. Cynthia Newby, *HIPAA for Allied Health Careers* (New York: McGraw-Hill Higher Education, 2009).

Chapter 12

Workplace Ethics

Many ethical dilemmas in health care are faced by patients and their families. Should a husband and father be taken off a ventilator and allowed to die? When should a do not resuscitate order be in place for an elderly patient with Alzheimer's disease? Is abortion permissible when the fetus has a serious genetic defect? Is it ethically permissible to use in vitro fertilization to overcome problems with infertility although a number of embryos will be lost?

This chapter will have a different focus. It will examine the ethical responsibilities of health care workers themselves and ethical dilemmas they may face *as employees* of a health care facility.

In this chapter you will learn about:

- the duty of a health care worker to provide care when risk is involved to himself/herself;
- an ethical principle for allocating time and services among patients;
- the ethics of health care workers "using their own judgment" in going against treatment orders for patients they are caring for;

- a health care worker's ethical responsibilities when a co-worker isn't doing his or her job.

Case Study

After the SARS (Severe Acute Respiratory Syndrome) outbreak in Toronto, the administration of Memorial Medical Center decides to be proactive in putting a policy into place to deal with epidemics. An ad hoc committee is established to draft a policy. Julia Dunn, a respiratory therapist, is appointed to the committee to represent allied health professionals.

The committee's task is to draft a policy that addresses issues such as working with public health and governmental officials, internal and external communications, education and training for staff, triage, allocation of vaccines and ventilators, and limiting access to the facility. (1) When it comes to the human resource issues that must be addressed, Julia feels ambivalent and a bit scared. She is pregnant. In the case of another outbreak of SARS, she knows that, as a respiratory therapist, she has special skills that would be much needed and could not be provided by other staff. At the same time, she wonders if she would be willing to come to work and risk being infected with a possibly fatal disease, especially while carrying a child.

The Duty to Care for Patients

In 1969 the U.S. Surgeon General William Stewart announced to Congress that "it is time to close the book on infectious diseases." (2) Subsequent events proved him to be very wrong in his judgment, most notably, the advent of HIV/AIDS and SARS. Outbreaks of infectious diseases can pose threats to health care workers themselves.

In August 2003 the World Health Organization announced that "20 percent of all persons known to have been infected with SARS were health care workers." (3) Of the forty-one people who died of SARS in Canada, three were health care professionals, as were six of the one hundred eighty persons who died of SARS in Taiwan. (3) Indeed, "Dr. Carolo Urbani of Medecins Sans Frontieres, who with others initially identified SARS as a new infectious disease in Hanoi, voluntarily quarantined himself and eventually died of SARS, leaving a widow and three children." (3) On the other hand, there were instances during the 2003 SARS outbreak in which some health care professionals "baulked at providing care to those infected with the unknown virus." (4) Sometimes "staffing became an issue in SARS wards and assessment centres; indeed, failure to report for duty during the outbreak resulted in the permanent dismissal of some hospital staff." (4) In sum, the SARS outbreak raised the question of the extent of a health care professional's duty to treat the victims of an outbreak of infectious disease, even at some substantial risk to the caregiver's own health and life. (3) The importance of this question is reinforced by the possibility of bioterrorism and predictions of an avian flu pandemic. (3)

The duty of health care professionals to provide care during an epidemic of an infectious disease is grounded ethically in several considerations.

- The principle of beneficence "recognizes and defines the special moral obligation on the part of HCPs [health care professionals] to further the welfare of patients and to advance patients' well-being." (4) (See chapter 1.)
- The ability and expertise of health care professionals to provide care is greater than that of the general public, thus increasing their obligation to provide care. (4)
- By freely choosing a profession devoted to care of the ill, health care professionals have consented to assuming greater than average risk. (4)
- In publicly funded health care systems, "there is a strong claim for a social contract between the HCP [health care professional] and society." (4) Specifically, "It is a reasonable and legitimate expectation by the public that HCPs will respond in an infectious disease emergency." (4)

On the other hand, there is recognition that an individual who is a health care professional likely functions in various roles—as spouse, parent, caregiver for relatives—and that these additional roles also carry ethical obligations. (4, 5) For example, health care workers have a duty to care for their own children during an epidemic by protecting them (and hence themselves) from infection. (5) Or, consider the following case of a health care professional...

> who is caring for an elderly parent in her home. Told to come to work in the face of a pandemic that could result in her being quarantined within the hospital for an indefinite period of time, and where her life would be put at risk, is she a bad person if she weighs her professional obligations against her duties to care for those who depend upon her at home?

According to McCullough's analysis, a health provider who could simply abandon her mother at home in the name of adhering to an abstract professional duty might not be the sort of human being we would wish to care for us . . . (3)

Moreover, health care professionals surely have "obligations to themselves and to their own health (particularly those with special vulnerabilities, such as a co-morbid condition)." (4)

In sum, health care professionals may have personal obligations to others and to themselves which conflict with their professional duty to provide care for patients during an outbreak of an infectious disease. This suggests that, while there is in general a duty on the part of health care workers to provide care to patients, this duty is limited and may have legitimate exceptions. (5) One strategy may be to allow certain cases in which a health care professional is considered exempt from coming to work during an epidemic of an infectious disease, perhaps being placed on furlough. (1) Short of this solution, policies may be put into place to reassign health care workers with special needs (e.g., female health care workers who are pregnant) to low risk duties, such as caring for patients who do not have the infectious disease or assuming administrative duties that do not involve patient care. (1) Or again, creative solutions might be developed for meeting both professional and personal duties. For example, an assistance program might be put into place to provide care at home for relatives of health care workers, making it more likely for them to come to work. (3) The discussion of how to resolve this conflict between professional and personal duties is ongoing. (3, 5)

Case Study

David Stock is a physical therapist who comes weekly to Stoneridge Manor to provide physical therapy services for its residents. Stoneridge is a multi-level facility for retired persons consisting of independent living apartments, assisted living units, and a nursing home unit.

David is currently providing physical therapy for three residents, Wanda Taylor, Fred Sullivan, and Mark Kohl. Before he visits these residents, he stops by the office of the director of nursing (DON) to get an update on their conditions.

Wanda is residing in the independent living apartments. The DON tells David that Wanda's daughter is making a trip today from another state to see her mother and bringing her children with her. They plan to take Wanda out to lunch. Because of the long driving distance, they're not sure exactly what time they will arrive that morning.

Fred is in the nursing home unit. The DON tells David that Fred has been experiencing considerable discomfort in his left leg for several days to the point of needing additional pain medication. The DON hopes that physical therapy will make him more comfortable.

Mark resides in the assisted living unit. Mark is the kind of person who has gone by a schedule all his life. He gets very upset when things get "off schedule," and this emotional stress aggravates his problem with high blood pressure. Mark is normally the first resident David treats, promptly at 11:00 a.m.

While David is having this conversation with the DON, the DON receives a call that a resident, Amanda Miller, has choked on a piece of hard candy she wasn't supposed to have in the first place, and that she has stopped breathing. Resuscitation is needed immediately. David has been trained in CPR.

To which resident should David give attention first?

■ ■ ■

Allocating Staff Time and Services among Patients

The time and services of health care workers are resources that must sometimes be allocated. Especially when there is a staffing shortage, health care workers may be faced with decisions about which patient should receive care first. Ethically, these allocation decisions involve *distributive justice,* the principle concerned with fairness in the distribution of benefits, burdens and resources. (See chapter 1.)

Philosophers have tried to spell out more concretely how benefits and resources are distributed fairly. One interpretation given to distributive justice is the *principle of equality,* according to which "everyone is to be treated the same in all respects." (6) More simply stated, this interpretation of distributive justice maintains that "everyone is entitled to the same size slice of the pie." (6) Another interpretation of distributive justice is the *principle of contribution,* according to which "everyone should get back that proportion of social goods that is the result of his or her productive labor." (6) If one person works twice as hard or long as a second, the first person should be entitled to twice as large a share in the benefits. (6) The interpretation of distributive justice that is most likely relevant to the situation of health care workers is the *principle of need:*

> The principle of need is an extension of the egalitarian principle of equal distribution. If goods are parceled out according to individual need, those who have greater needs will receive a greater share. However, the outcome will be one of equality. Since the basic needs of everyone will be met, everyone will end up at the same level. The treatment of individuals will be equal, in this respect, even though the proportion of goods they receive will not be. (6)

Thus, if two (or more) patients need attention, a health care worker should prioritize his or her services and time according to which patient has the greater (greatest) need.

Let us apply the principle of need to the decisions David Stock has to make. First, David has to decide between giving physical therapy to Wanda, Fred, and Mark (the reason he came to Stoneridge Manor) and administering CPR to Amanda, the resident who choked on a piece of candy. Amanda is in a life-threatening situation while Wanda, Fred, and Mark are not. Clearly, the resident who choked and needs resuscitation has the greatest need. If no one else who is adequately trained in CPR is immediately available, David should respond to Amanda first.

The problem is that many decisions about allocating time and services are not this clear cut. Suppose that the DON can attend to Amanda, allowing David to proceed with the physical therapy services for which he came to Stoneridge Manor. Mark is probably already upset that David is late to administer his physical therapy, and this is not good for his blood pressure. While Mark is experiencing emotional distress, Fred has been experiencing serious physical discomfort. Physical therapy may well help relieve the discomfort he has been experiencing for several days. And on the other hand, if David does not attend to Wanda right away, her daughter may come to take her to lunch before David can get to her. If Wanda misses her physical therapy entirely, this is likely to result in physical discomfort for her later in the week. Which of these residents should David attend to first? Whose need is the greatest?

If Fred is presently experiencing serious discomfort, we would likely judge his need to be the greatest. On the other hand, if his discomfort is being adequately managed through pain medication, he could probably wait a bit to have his physical therapy administered.

We might then consider the needs of Wanda to be the most urgent. After all, it may be a case of Wanda receiving therapy now or forgoing it entirely for that week. Mark will eventually receive his therapy, the only question is when.

At the same, Mark's emotional distress cannot be totally discounted. Indeed, this may aggravate his high blood pressure. Mark, too, has a real need.

In this case, a solution might be found to meet the needs of both Wanda and Mark. Before seeing Wanda, perhaps David could stop into Mark's room to calm him down by explaining the needs of other residents that require his attention, and reassuring him that he will be back to administer his therapy as soon as he is able.

Case Study

Julie Ames works as a dietitian at Spring Valley Home. Part of her job is making sure that dietary restrictions for particular residents are observed. Because of heart problems, George Mason's doctor has put him on a low-fat, low sodium diet. George usually cooperates without too much complaint, but he loves sweet corn and "just can't eat it without some salt." Spring Valley always has a picnic for residents on the Fourth of July, and this year a local farmer—in fact, a friend of George—has donated a truckload of sweet corn to the home for the picnic. Julie knows that George will feel left out and hurt if he isn't served sweet corn, especially since it comes from a personal friend. She also knows that if George is served the sweet corn plain, he will raise a fuss with the staff about getting some salt. A conflict between George and the staff during the picnic will ruin the day for both him and the staff. Julie decides to slip two packets of salt onto George's tray. After all, George's doctor will never know, and this one breach of his diet shouldn't harm him.

■ ■ ■

Staff Who "Use Their Own Judgment"

In this case, a staff member of a health care facility takes it upon herself to do something for a resident that directly goes against the orders of a physician. The staff member makes the judgment that the resident's health will not be harmed by going against the physician's orders. Ethically, is it permissible for staff to act in this way?

Some would approach this case not by looking at the behavior of staff, but rather, by focusing on residents and their autonomy. Allowing a person to direct the course of his or her own life is a value much emphasized in contemporary health care ethics. Thus, some would argue that the proper course of action is to explain to George the possible consequences for his heart condition of using salt, but to allow him to make the decision whether he wishes to take those risks. Once health care providers have informed George of the risks and are confident that he understands them and is mentally competent to make decisions, then both the physician and the nursing home staff should abide by George's wishes, even if they personally disagree with his choice. If George wants salt for his sweet corn, he should have it! (7)

However, not everyone would place such an exclusive emphasis on patient autonomy. They would point out that health care providers have a duty of *nonmaleficence,* a duty to prevent harm from coming to patients. In the case of George, autonomy and nonmaleficence may be in conflict. (See chapter 1.) In others words, there may be a conflict between what George wants to do in terms of eating and what his doctor believes should be done to prevent further harm to his already fragile health.

The question can be raised whether Julie the dietitian violated the ethical duty of nonmaleficence in providing salt for George. She "used her own judgment" in believing that George would not be harmed by her action. But can she really be so sure that she has the professional knowledge to make these assessments on her own?

Further, Julie's behavior is ethically questionable because it is deceptive. In slipping two packets of salt onto George's tray, Julie believes that "George's doctor will never know."

If staff member Julie questioned the wisdom of an absolute prohibition of salt seasoning for George, it would have been more appropriate for her to raise this question with her supervisor, with George's physician, or at the care conference for George. Bringing this question out into the open would provide the opportunity to discuss whether occasional indulgences in salt seasoning would in fact be harmful to George's health. After discussion, perhaps George's physician would agree to occasional indulgences.

Case Study

Rhonda Lewis is an RN who has worked for ten years at Spring Valley Home. She is known as a good worker and as someone who is very conscientious. Rhonda has some concerns about Jerry Miles who comes every week to administer physical therapy to some of the residents of Spring Valley Home. Several times, she has smelled alcohol on Jerry's breath. On one occasion she walked into George Mason's room and found Jerry helping him with exercises for his legs. The problem is that George didn't need these exercises. Jerry was supposed to give them to the man in the room next to George's. George wasn't at all hurt by this mistake, but Rhonda wonders how often this kind of mistake is occurring. Another resident, Henry Thompson, has complained to her that Jerry has skipped him on several occasions. And when Henry doesn't get his exercises, he gets stiff and experiences some difficulty in walking. Rhonda wonders what she should do. She has always believed that co-workers should not "rat" on each other. And she knows how difficult it is to get outside health care workers to provide services at a nursing home, especially on a weekly basis. What will the residents of Spring Valley Home do if they lose Jerry?

■ ■ ■

Problems with the Job Performance of Co-Workers

In this case, Rhonda is concerned about the job performance of a co-worker, Jerry, who comes to Spring Valley Home to administer physical therapy to some of the residents. She has caught one mistake Jerry made on the job, giving exercises to the wrong resident. In this case, the mistake didn't cause the resident any harm. But if this sort of mistake occurs again, it is possible that a resident could suffer from the unneeded exercises. Also, Jerry has caused discomfort to another resident on several occasions by forgetting about his therapy altogether. In addition, Rhonda worries about the fact that she has smelled alcohol on Jerry's breath several times. She knows that alcohol can impair performance and cause someone to make mistakes.

The ethical duty of nonmaleficence tells Rhonda that she must act to prevent harm from coming to the residents of Spring Valley Home. (See chapter 1.) The situation with Jerry presents the potential for harm. Therefore, Rhonda cannot just let this situation slip by, but is morally obligated to take action.

Rhonda has strong feelings that co-workers should not "rat" on each other. Perhaps, then, the first step is for Rhonda to confront Jerry himself with her concerns about his job performance. Is it the case that Jerry has made mistakes and been forgetful because of a stressful situation within his own family that is only temporary? Or are his mistakes and forgetfulness due to a more enduring problem? What is the cause of Jerry's apparent alcohol abuse? On his own, will Jerry decide to get appropriate professional help if needed?

In her job, Rhonda's first obligation is to the residents of Spring Valley Home and to promoting their welfare and protecting them from harm. If Rhonda's conversation with Jerry does not result in a change of job performance, or if Rhonda does not feel comfortable about having such a conversation with Jerry, then she has an obligation to report this situation to her supervisor. While she may not want to "rat" on Jerry, her obligation to prevent harm to residents takes precedence over her feelings.

CHAPTER SUMMARY

Key Terms and Concepts

principle of patient autonomy: self-determination; the right of a patient to make the final decision in matters pertaining to his or her own life and health care.

principle of beneficence: the ethical duty to act for the benefit and welfare of others.

principle of nonmaleficence: the ethical duty not to inflict harm on others.

principle of distributive justice: fairness in the distribution of benefits, burdens, and resources.

principle of need: an interpretation of distributive justice giving priority in the distribution of resources to those with the greatest need.

Key Points

- In general, health care workers have a professional duty to provide care for patients, even in cases (such as an outbreak of an infectious disease) posing risk to their own health and life. However, this duty may be limited by personal obligations of the health care workers.
- Because of staffing shortages, health care workers may have to make decisions about which patients to help and which ones must have care postponed, at least temporarily. Ethically, a guiding principle is the *principle of need*, directing health care workers to prioritize their time and services according to which patient has the greater (greatest) need.
- Health care workers have a duty of nonmaleficence; that is, a duty to act in ways that prevent harm from coming to patients. Health care workers should be cautious about "using their own judgment" in ways that go against the course of treatment prescribed for a patient. If a health care worker

believes that the prescribed course of treatment is not in the patient's best interests, he or she should raise this issue with a supervisor, with the patient's physician, or at a care conference.
- When a health care worker observes job performance problems with co-workers (for example, treatment mistakes, failure to do the job at all, impairment due to substance abuse) which may bring harm to patients, the duty of nonmaleficence requires him or her to take preventive action. This may mean alerting supervisors to the job performance problem.

FOR FURTHER DISCUSSION

1. In this chapter we have discussed the extreme case of a health care worker's obligation to come to work in the event of an epidemic of an infectious disease. But consider the following scenario:

   > Brigid O'Connor is director of radiologic services at St. Luke's Hospital. Among her duties, she is responsible for seeing that there is adequate staffing. On several occasions, she has called in Sally Furtweiler, one of the technologists in the department. Sally frequently telephones at the last minute to say that she cannot come to work that day. On one occasion, she said she had car trouble. On another occasion, she had an emergency dental appointment. On more than one occasion, she's said she cannot come to work because of a sick child or because of bad weather. Then there was the time Sally didn't come in because her sister came to visit from California. Brigid is tempted to fire Sally for excessive absenteeism, but she doesn't do so because of the staffing shortage health care facilities in that geographical area are experiencing. Brigid reasons that having Sally work part of the time is better than nothing!
   >
   > However, Sally's absence from work unexpectedly and frequently presents a staffing problem. Roy Taylor works with Sally on the same shift, and Roy has complained to Brigid several times about not being able to take care of all the patients properly when Sally is absent.
   >
   > On one occasion, when Roy was the only radiographer on duty, he took an x-ray which showed the patient to have an enlarged heart. When this was reported to the patient, she became very distressed. This patient has problems with high blood pressure, and

her anxiety over the results of the x-ray only aggravated her problem. Further diagnostic testing showed that the x-ray picture had been faulty, probably because Roy was in such a hurry to take it.

On that same occasion, the fact that "one person had to do the work of two" caused a delay in Roy responding to a request for x-rays in the emergency room. This, in turn, caused a delay in treating the patient.

We would all agree that there are emergency situations that make absence from work necessary and justified. However, it seems that Sally Furtweiler is not taking her duty to come to work seriously enough.

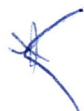

In what circumstances do you think it is legitimate for a health care worker to decide not to come to work? Is bad weather a legitimate reason? Caring for a sick child? Personal illness? An emergency dental appointment?

Hint: Try using the utilitarian ethical theory in working through these questions, looking at the consequences for everyone who will be affected by the course of action. (See chapter 1.)

2. Pam Hays is a respiratory therapist at Westridge Hospital. Because of an outbreak of flu, she is the only respiratory therapist currently on duty. Her two co-workers have called in sick.

John Wright has been hospitalized for emphysema, but is scheduled to be released this morning. Pam is scheduled to give him therapy at 9:00 a.m. before he leaves for home.

When Pam is on her way to see John, she is paged to go to the emergency room (ER). Instinctively she does this, where she is asked to set up a ventilator for a patient who has just been brought to the ER. While she is doing this, a nurse tells her that a mother has just come to the ER with a child who has cystic fibrosis. The mother is concerned that the therapy she did at home that morning with her son did not adequately clear the mucus from his lungs. She has taken time off from work to bring her son to the emergency room, but needs to return to work as soon as possible.

Pam, a mother herself, sympathizes with this woman's concerns about her son and appreciates the time constraints she is under with respect to her job. At the same time, Pam knows that she has the scheduled appointment with Mr. Wright, and that his wife is coming to take him home shortly. Pam is faced with a dilemma: Should she next attend to the boy with cystic fibrosis, or to Mr. Wright?

In your judgment, whom should Pam see next? What are the reasons behind your judgment?

3. Ted Collins is on the dietary staff at Spring Valley Home. He smokes heavily. He doesn't smoke in the facility itself, but whenever he gets a break from his work in the kitchen, he goes outside and lights up. A co-worker, Jill Pierce, is upset with Ted for doing this. She tells him that residents who are walking or sitting outdoors can see him smoke, and that this tempts residents who are restricted from smoking for health reasons. Jill tells her supervisor that Ted should be made to give up smoking entirely while at work.

   - *Is this situation different from the case of Jerry Miles, who showed up at Spring Valley Home to administer physical therapy with alcohol on his breath?*
   - *Jill's complaints to her supervisor would be legitimate and would fall under the duty of nonmaleficence if Ted's behavior at work poses a threat of harm to the residents. Can a case be made that Ted is harming residents by his smoking?*

4. Suppose that you are asked to serve on an ad hoc committee to develop specific criteria for the annual staff evaluation process. What specific standards would you suggest for the areas of absence from work, following treatment directives for patients, and handling job performance problems with co-workers? And why would you suggest these particular standards?

References

1. Centers for Disease Control and Prevention, *HHS Pandemic Influenza Plan Supplement 3 Healthcare Planning*, http://www.hhs.gov/pandemicflu/plan/sup3.html. Accessed March 2009.
2. Daniel K. Sokol, "Doctors' first duty: Professional or personal?" *International Herald Tribune* (October 21, 2005), http://www.iht.com/articles/2005/10/21/opinion/edsokol.php. Accessed March 2009.
3. Howard Brody and Eric N. Avery, "Medicine's Duty to Treat Pandemic Illness Solidarity and Vulnerability," *Hastings Center Report* 39/1 (January-February 2009): 40-48.
4. Carly Ruderman, C. Shawn Tracy, Cecile M. Bensimon, Mark Bernstein, Laura Hawryluck, Randi Zlotnik Shaul, Ross EG Upshur, "On pandemics and

the duty to care: whose duty? whose care?" *BMC Medical Ethics* 7/5 (2006). http://www.biomedcentral.com/1472-6939/7/5. Accessed March 2009.
5. Daniel K. Sokol, "Virulent Epidemics and Scope of Healthcare Workers' Duty of Care," *Emerging Infectious Diseases* 12/8 (August 2006), http://www.cdc.gov/ncidod/ EID/vol12no08/06-0360.htm. Accessed March 2009.
6. "Principles of Distributive Justice" in Ronald Munson (ed.), *Intervention and Reflection: Basic Issues in Medical Ethics,* 8th ed. (Belmont, CA: Thomson Wadsworth, 2008).
7. "Beyond the Call of Duty: A Nurse's Aide Uses Her Judgment" in Rosalie Kane & Arthur L. Caplan (eds.), *Everyday Ethics: Resolving Dilemmas in Nursing Home Life* (New York: Springer, 1990).

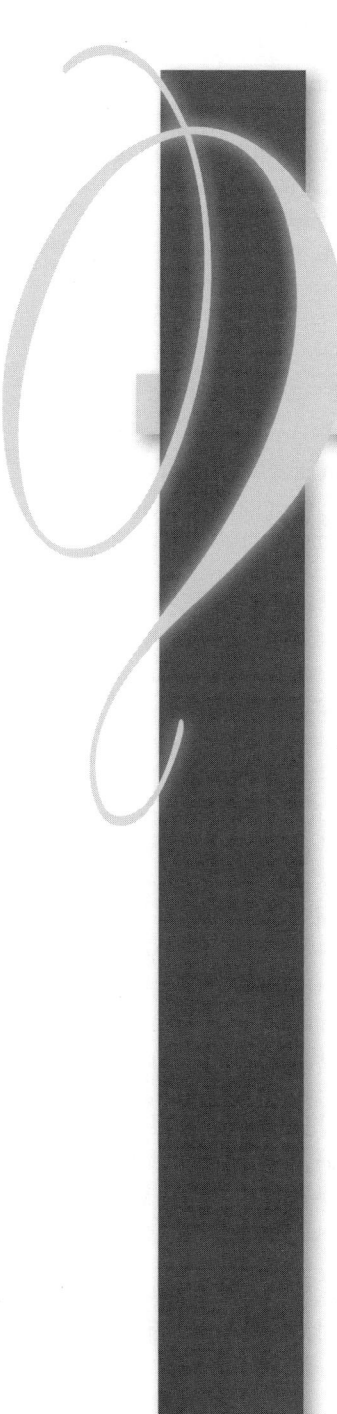

Chapter 13

Ethical and Religious Objections to Health Care Practices

Health care treatments and interventions can be ethically and religiously controversial. The abortion debate in the United States is a prime example of this. Some people favor assisted suicide, whereas others are opposed to it on ethical and religious grounds. Some have objections in conscience to such practices as in vitro fertilization and the freezing of embryos. While most people in American society take blood transfusions for granted, Jehovah's Witnesses refuse them on religious grounds.

Patients will bring their ethical and religious values with them when seeking health care services. Similarly, health care workers also have personal beliefs about what is right and wrong to do.

In this chapter you will learn about:

- the right of an adult patient to refuse a medical treatment on ethical or religious grounds;

- the scope of parental authority to refuse a medical treatment for a child because of ethical or religious objections to it;
- the right of a health care worker to be excused from participating in a treatment or course of action to which s/he has ethical or religious objections.

Case Study

Rebecca Stanton, 43, is an outpatient at the cancer treatment center of St. Margaret's Medical Center. She is undergoing radiation treatments for a small cancerous tumor in her stomach. The prospects for the cancer going into remission look good. Extensive examination also indicates a pre-leukemic blood condition, but Rebecca's physician is confident that this can be successfully treated with monthly blood transfusions.

When Rebecca is approached about beginning the blood transfusions, she unqualifiedly refuses. She states that she is a Jehovah's Witness, and that her religion does not permit blood transfusions. She says that she will put her faith in God. "If God wants me to continue to live," she states, "I will recover without the blood transfusions."

St. Margaret's is a Catholic-sponsored facility, a religious tradition that accepts the practice of blood transfusions. The oncology staff at St. Margaret's cannot understand how there can be *religious* reasons for refusing a blood transfusion that clearly will be beneficial to someone's health.

Rebecca has taken a special liking to one radiation therapist, Barbara Baxter. Several members of the oncology staff ask Barbara to talk to Rebecca about the transfusions. Barbara poses to Rebecca a situation in which she thinks it will be impossible for Rebecca to condemn transfusions. "Think back to the time when your son was just five years old," Barbara tells Rebecca, "and was injured in an automobile accident. Suppose that your son had been so severely injured that he would die unless he had a blood transfusion. As a mother, wouldn't you have wanted the transfusion to save your son's life?" To Barbara's surprise, Rebecca calmly replies that she could have accepted her son's death as God's will.

At this point, Barbara Baxter and several other staff members ask to meet with the hospital's ethics committee to help them deal with this baffling situation.

■ ■ ■

Objections to Health Care Practices by Patients and Families

Perhaps the classic case of a religious objection to a medical practice is the refusal of blood transfusions by Jehovah's Witnesses. This refusal is based on Old Testament texts, such as Genesis 9:4, Leviticus 3:17 and 7:26, and Acts 15:28-29, which forbid "partaking of any blood." (1, 2)

A famous court case involving the refusal of blood transfusions by a Jehovah's Witness is *In re Brooks Estate* from the state of Illinois. In May, 1964, Bernice Brooks was in McNeal General Hospital in Chicago, suffering from a peptic ulcer. She was attended by Dr. Gilbert Demange, and had informed him repeatedly during a two-year period prior to her hospitalization that her religious beliefs prevented her from receiving blood transfusions. In fact, Mrs. Brooks and her husband signed a document releasing Dr. Demange and the hospital from all civil liability that might result from a failure to administer blood transfusions to Mrs. Brooks. In spite of this, Dr. Demange, together with several assistant State's attorneys and the attorney for the public guardian of Cook County, Illinois, appeared before the probate division of the circuit court with a petition by the public guardian requesting appointment of the guardian as conservator of Bernice Brooks. Further, the petition requested an order authorizing the conservator to consent to administration of blood to Mrs. Brooks. The court appointed the conservator, and a blood transfusion was administered to Mrs. Brooks. (3)

This situation involved a conflict between what the patient wanted (namely, no blood transfusions) and what the physician felt obligated to do for the welfare of the patient. Ethically speaking, this situation involved a conflict between *patient autonomy* and the health care professional's duty of *beneficence*. (See chapter 1.)

The Illinois court made the following judgment in this case:

> ... It seems to be clearly established that the First Amendment of the United States Constitution, as extended to the individual States by the Fourteenth Amendment to that Constitution, protects the absolute right of every individual to freedom in his religious belief and the exercise thereof, subject only to the qualification that the exercise thereof may be properly limited by governmental action where such exercise endangers, clearly and presently, the public health, welfare or morals.
>
> ... No overt or affirmative act of appellants offers any clear and present danger to society—we have only a governmental agency compelling conduct offensive to appellant's religious principles. Even though we may consider appellant's beliefs unwise, foolish or ridiculous, in the absence of an overriding danger to society we may not permit interference

therewith in the form of a conservatorship established in the waning hours of her life for the sole purpose of compelling her to accept medical treatment forbidden by her religious principles and previously refused by her with full knowledge of the probable consequences. In the final analysis, what has happened here involves a judicial attempt to decide what course of action is best for a particular individual, notwithstanding that individual's contrary views based upon religious convictions. Such action cannot be constitutionally countenanced. (3)

The Illinois court took the position that an individual's religious freedom must be respected and can only be limited when the person's behavior threatens harm to society. Thus, Mrs. Brooks had the right to refuse blood transfusions on religious grounds, and it was wrong for a conservator to have been appointed to force blood transfusions on her.

In the case of Mrs. Brooks, the Illinois court came down on the side of patient autonomy. Several arguments might be put forward to support giving priority to individual autonomy in this case. (See chapter 1.)

First, patients other than Jehovah's Witnesses can and do make the choice not to follow their physician's recommendations. In one study, "19% of patients at teaching hospitals refused at least one treatment or procedure, even though 15% of such refusals were potentially life endangering." (4) Generalizing this point, refusing a medical procedure on religious grounds can be seen as one instance of the phenomenon of patient choice regarding medical treatments.

Moreover, there are other cases in which therapies have to be altered to accommodate special circumstances, such as hypertension, severe allergy to antibiotics, or the unavailability of certain costly equipment. (4) Analogously, when a patient objects to a particular medical treatment on religious grounds, health care providers "are being asked to manage the medical or surgical problem in harmony with the patient's choice and conscience." (4)

Finally, health care providers should keep in mind the psychological damage that may be inflicted on a patient by forcing her to undergo a medical treatment against her conscience:

> If a court forced an abhorrent treatment on you, how might this affect your conscience and the vital element of your will to live? Dr. Konrad Drebinger wrote: "It would certainly be a misguided form of medical ambition that would lead one to force a patient to accept a given therapy, overruling his conscience, so as to treat him physically but dealing his psyche a mortal blow." (2)

In other words, the focus should be on treating "the whole person." (5)

The case study of Rebecca Stanton hypothesizes a scenario in which her son would need a blood transfusion after being seriously injured in an auto accident. This scenario differs in one important respect from the case of Mrs. Brooks. Rebecca's son is only five years old, and the decision to forgo a blood transfusion would be made by his parents. While it is recognized that a mentally competent adult patient who has been adequately informed of the potential advantages and risks of a proposed treatment does have the right to refuse it, even when the best medical opinion deems it essential to save the patient's life (6, 7), it is another issue whether parents can legitimately make this decision for a child who is incapable of deciding for himself. (8)

While there is a presumption in favor of parental decision-making authority for their children, that parental authority is not absolute. Legally, children fall under the *parens patriae* power of the state as persons unable to protect themselves. (9) In the exercise of this power, the state may step in before parental decisions "become operative to ensure that the choices made are not so detrimental to a child's interests as to amount to neglect and abuse." (9) Parents are considered to be "under obligation to provide minor children with the necessities of life, which includes medical care deemed necessary to prevent children's deaths." (10) And, "if any or all of this is not performed, the principles of law override professed religious convictions of the parents." (10) As stated by the Superior Court of the State of Illinois:

> Parents may be free to become martyrs themselves. It does not follow, however, that they are free in identical circumstances to make martyrs of their children before they have reached an age of full and legal discretion, when they can make that choice for themselves. Laws, while they cannot interfere with religious belief and opinion, may be constitutionally appropriate for interfering with religious practices. (11)

If a child of Jehovah's Witnesses requires a blood transfusion, a court could intervene and appoint a legal guardian other than the child's parents who would authorize the transfusion. (11) Indeed, one court "took the view that a judicially ordered blood transfusion could properly be administered to a pregnant patient, when such was necessary to save her life, even though she and her husband had refused to authorize transfusions because of their religious beliefs, upon the grounds that it would be justified in the interest of protecting the unborn child . . . ". (11)

In sum, St. Margaret's Medical Center would be obliged to treat the cases of Rebecca Stanton and of her son differently. While staff could try to persuade Rebecca to have needed blood transfusions, they would be required to respect her wishes to decline them if that were her ultimate decision. On the other hand, if Rebecca refused needed blood transfusions for her son, the staff could pursue legal action, asking for a legal guardian other than his parents to be appointed to make the medical treatment decisions. (6)

What has been said about the case of Jehovah's Witnesses and refusal of blood transfusions would apply to other cases of religious objections to health care treatments and interventions. For example, it would apply to those who reject "standard" medical treatment in favor of faith-healing services.

Case Study

Terry Welsh is a new respiratory therapist at St. Margaret's Medical Center. He is very active in a local pro-life group. He has strong feelings that it is morally wrong to withhold or withdraw life-sustaining treatments. This is, he believes, just a way of "getting rid of people who are difficult or whose care is expensive." He is also against advance directives because they allow forgoing life-sustaining treatments. In fact, he has a stack of pamphlets warning against advance directives, and he has been known to pass them out to patients and families at the hospital.

John Springer is in the final stages of Alzheimer's disease, and has been transferred from a nursing home to St. Margaret's because he has developed pneumonia. Antibiotic treatment and ventilator support with supplemental oxygen are initiated. Several days pass, but John does not appear to improve.

A durable power of attorney for health care executed by John names his wife, Louise, as his proxy decision maker. After talking with their children, Louise tells John's physician that she wants the antibiotics and ventilator support stopped. Alzheimer's disease is a terminal condition, she says, and John is at the stage where he can no longer enjoy life because he is bedridden and suffering from severe dementia. "John would never want to live like this," she states. She believes it is time that the natural dying process should be allowed to take its course. After all, pneumonia is "the old person's friend." John's physician agrees with her.

Terry Welsh is instructed by John's physician to disconnect the ventilator. However, Terry tells his supervisor that John's family and physician are "killing him" by not administering antibiotics and by withdrawing the ventilator, and that his conscience will not allow him to be a part of this affair. "On moral grounds," he tells his supervisor, "I can no longer be involved in John's case."

■ ■ ■

Objections of Conscience by Health Care Workers

Health care workers may sometimes be asked to perform a procedure or participate in a course of action to which they personally object on ethical or religious grounds. A common case is the participation of health care workers in abortion procedures. But this is not the only kind of situation in which objections of conscience can arise. In this case, Terry, a respiratory therapist, firmly believes it is morally wrong to withhold or withdraw life-sustaining treatments, and refuses to participate in the care of John Springer, a patient with pneumonia from whom antibiotics and ventilator support are to be withdrawn by the choice of his proxy decision maker. In Terry's mind, an action on his part of disconnecting John's ventilator would be participating in the process of deliberately causing a patient's death.

It is recognized that health care facilities can legitimately refuse to provide what a patient (or his proxy decision maker) may want. As stated by the Special Committee on Biomedical Ethics of the American Hospital Association, "Generally, a hospital may refuse to provide a service to a patient if the procedure is inappropriate to its mission (for example, therapeutic abortion, artificial insemination)." (12) Similarly, the federal *Patient Self-Determination Act* on advance directives contains a conscience clause. With respect to complying with the directives set out by a patient in a living will or durable power of attorney for health care, no facility is required to act contrary to its own mission and ethical values. However, a health care facility must have clearly written policies specifying the limits on the procedures it will perform, and make this information available to its clients. (13)

Similarly, it is recognized that health care workers have a right to refuse to participate in procedures and courses of action to which they personally have ethical or religious objections. As stated by the Special Committee on Biomedical Ethics of the American Hospital Association:

> If a patient chooses a course of treatment that is not acceptable to the attending physician or other health care professionals, those individuals may withdraw from the case, as long as doing so does not amount to legal abandonment. If a suitably qualified alternative physician or health care professional willing to comply with the patient's preference is available, transfer to the care of that individual should be offered to the patient. (12)

Thus, if Terry believes it is ethically wrong to forgo life-sustaining treatments (in this case, antibiotics and ventilator support for pneumonia), he should be allowed to withdraw from being involved in the care of John Springer, with another respiratory therapist taking his place. However, there are several provisos for this concession to Terry.

First, Terry has an obligation to make known his treatment refusal "in advance and in time for other appropriate arrangements to be made" for the care of the patient. (14) Terry knows that he has ethical objections in principle to any case of withholding or withdrawing a life-sustaining treatment from a patient. And he knows that instances of withholding or withdrawing life-sustaining treatments are likely to occur in a hospital setting. He has an obligation to let his supervisor know about his ethical stance *before* he is faced with the case of John Springer. After all, the hospital will have to make arrangements for another respiratory therapist to take Terry's place in caring for John. If Terry just suddenly announces his ethical objections to participating in withdrawing the ventilator, the hospital may not be able to locate a substitute respiratory therapist and John's dying process may be prolonged and his wife may be distressed.

Second, Terry must make sure that his refusal to participate in withdrawing the ventilator is based on accurate and complete information. (14, 15) Terry believes that withholding or withdrawing life-sustaining treatments is just a way of "getting rid of people who are difficult or whose care is expensive." But does he really understand what people's motivation can be for forgoing life-sustaining treatments? The motivation of John's wife seems to be that she does not want to prolong her husband's suffering, and that John himself would not want to live completely bedridden and with severe dementia. Does Terry recognize the emotional strain John's wife may be experiencing in "letting go" of her husband? Does Terry understand that there is a difference between forgoing life-sustaining treatments and involuntary euthanasia (which may be an attempt to "get rid of people")? Is he familiar with what ethicists and religious denominations are saying about the permissibility of forgoing life-sustaining treatments? In sum, before Terry can legitimately voice an objection of conscience to participating in withdrawing the ventilator, he has an obligation to become factually and ethically informed about withholding and withdrawing life-sustaining treatments.

Suppose that Terry persists in his belief that it is ethically wrong to withhold or withdraw life-sustaining treatments. He may have to consider changing his place of employment. It is undoubtedly a policy of St. Margaret's Medical Center to allow patients to forgo life-sustaining treatments. If it becomes a frequent occurrence that a substitute worker has to be found for Terry because of his objections of conscience and if this proves difficult for Terry's supervisor to do, then Terry's job performance may be called into question. In this case, it may be best for Terry to seek employment at a facility holding ethical views more similar to his own. It is nothing new to say that there may be a price to pay for adhering to one's ethical principles.

CHAPTER SUMMARY

Key Terms and Concepts

principle of autonomy: self-determination; the right of a patient to make the final decision in matters pertaining to his or her own life and health care.
principle of beneficence: the duty to act for the benefit and welfare of others.

Key Points

- An adult patient who is mentally competent and who has been adequately informed of the potential advantages and risks of a medical treatment does have the right to refuse it. The grounds for refusal may be ethical or religious, even if these beliefs are not accepted by other people.
- Parents cannot make the same kinds of decisions about refusing medical treatment for their children that they can make for themselves. Under the *parens patriae* power of the state, types of medical treatment can be legally mandated for children even though the parents find them ethically or religiously objectionable.
- A health care facility can legitimately refuse to provide to a patient a service that goes against the facility's mission and ethical values.
- Health care workers have a right to refuse to participate in procedures and courses of action that go against their ethical principles and religious beliefs. However, this refusal should be made known in advance and in time for other arrangements to be made for patient care.
- Objections of conscience are responsibly made by health care workers only if they are based on accurate and complete information about the facts of the case and about relevant ethical principles.
- For the sake of satisfactory job performance, a health care worker who has ethical or religious objections to a procedure or course of action allowed by the facility's policies may be faced with the decision of seeking employment at another facility.

FOR FURTHER DISCUSSION

1. Are there any religious groups (e.g., Christian Scientists) in your geographical area whose beliefs may affect their acceptance of "standard" health care practices, procedures, and technologies? How much do you know about the beliefs of such groups?
2. Are there any procedures or courses of action in caring for patients that you yourself find ethically objectionable? Religiously objectionable? If so, what are the grounds on which you find them objectionable?

   Do you think that your ethical or religious views may cause you to run into any problems in your job or role in health care? Can you think of means to accommodate your objections of conscience while still doing your job or fulfilling your role satisfactorily?
3. Courts have the power to arrange for medical treatments for children even though their parents find them ethically or religiously objectionable. Do you think that courts ought to have this power, or that parental decision-making authority on behalf of their children should be absolute? How would you feel if legal measures were taken to initiate a medical treatment on one of your children against your wishes?

References

1. Orville N. Griese, *Catholic Identity in Health Care: Principles and Practice* (Braintree, MA: Pope John Center, 1987).
2. Jehovah's Witnesses Official Web Site, "You Have the Right to Choose," http://www.watchtower.org/e/hb/article_04.htm. Accessed February 2009.
3. Emory C. Underwood, "From *In re Brooks Estate*" in J. Katz (ed.), *Experimentation with Human Beings* (New York: Russell Sage Foundation, 1972).
4. J. Lowell Dixon, "Blood: Whose Choice and Whose Conscience?" *New York State Journal of Medicine* 88 (1988): 463-4.
5. "Jehovah's Witnesses: The Surgical/Ethical Challenge," *Journal of the American Medical Association* 246/21 (Nov. 27, 1981): 2471-2.
6. Laurance T. Wren, "Status of the Law on Medical and Religious Conflicts in Blood Transfusions," *Arizona Medicine* 24 (October 1967): 970-73.

7. David H. Wilson, "Patients' Wishes Must Be Accepted," *British Medical Journal* 308 (28 May 1994): 1424.
8. Baruch Brody, Commentary on "Faith Healing for Childhood Leukemia" in Bette-Jane Crigger (ed.), *Cases in Bioethics: Selections from the Hastings Center Report*, 3rd ed. (New York: St. Martin's Press, 1998).
9. President's Commission for the Study of Ethical Problems in Medicine and Biomedical and Behavioral Research, *Deciding to Forego Life-Sustaining Treatment* (March 1983; reprint New York: Concern for Dying).
10. J.W. Holloway, Jr., "Blood Transfusions—Jehovah's Witnesses," *Journal of the American Medical Association* 163 (1957): 660, quoted in 11 below.
11. George Thomas, Robert W. Edmark & Thomas Jones, "Issues Involved with Surgery of Jehovah's Witnesses," *The American Surgeon* 34/7 (July 1968): 542-43.
12. Special Committee on Biomedical Ethics, *Values in Conflict Resolving Ethical Issues in Hospital Care* (Chicago: American Hospital Association, 1985).
13. Catholic Health Association of the United States, *The Patient Self-Determination Act* (St. Louis: Catholic Health Association of the United States, 1991).
14. Ellen W. Bernal & Patricia S. Hoover, Commentary on "The Nurse's Appeal to Conscience" in Bette-Jane Crigger (ed.), *Cases in Bioethics: Selections from the Hastings Center Report*, 3rd ed. (New York: St. Martin's Press, 1998).
15. Mila Ann Aroskar, Commentary on "The Nurse's Appeal to Conscience" in Bette-Jane Crigger (ed.), *Cases in Bioethics Selections from the Hastings Center Report*, 3rd ed. (New York: St. Martin's Press, 1998).

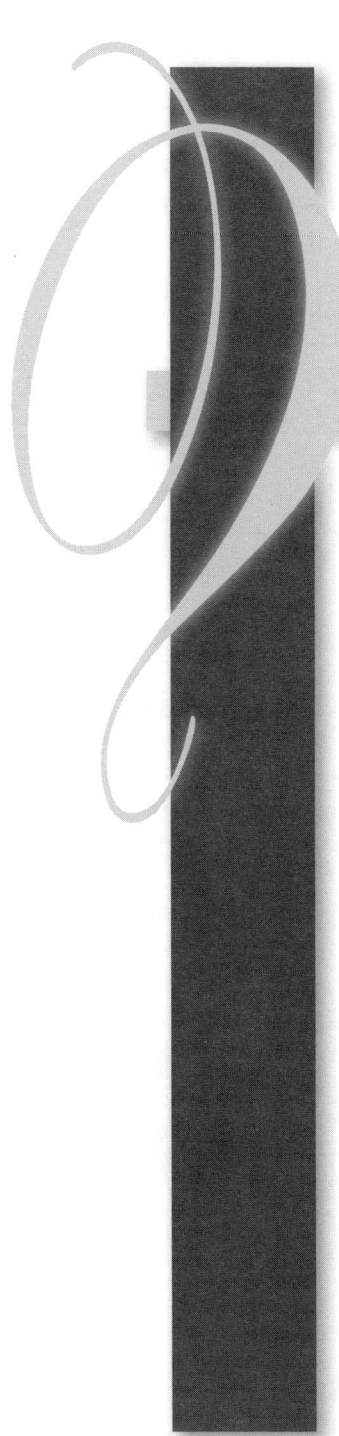

Chapter 14

Multicultural Perspectives in Health Care

More and more it is being recognized that some principles of American health care ethics may not be universally accepted. For example, Western health care ethics "endorses certain practices such as informed consent, disclosure of diagnosis and prognosis, and termination of treatment under certain conditions of terminal illness." (1) These practices, in turn, "reflect certain values widely held in Western culture: the autonomy of the individual person, the imperatives favoring truthfulness and open communication, and the realistic assessment of the efficacy of medical care." (1) However, health care workers who are trained in these practices and values may encounter patients and families from various cultures and subcultures who "react negatively or paradoxically to these practices." (1) In such cases conflicts can arise between health care providers and patients and their families.

In this chapter you will learn about:

- the practice of telling the truth about her condition to a patient who is terminally ill;
- cultures with different views than American bioethics on truth telling to the terminally ill, patient autonomy, pain management, and the practice of informed consent;
- ways in which health care providers can deal with multiculturalism;
- the competing theories of ethical relativism and ethical objectivism.

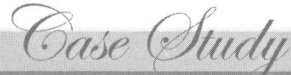

Case Study

The Pleasant Hill Care Center is located in a Midwestern community that has recently seen an influx of Asian residents. This is because of a faculty and student exchange program established by a local college.

Mr. Chang has come with his family to the United States from China to teach at the college. Mr. Chang's mother, 84, accompanied them to the United States because she is a widow and in poor health. In fact, multiple health problems and general physical debilitation soon led to her placement in the Pleasant Hill Care Center.

The adjustment to the nursing home has been very difficult for Mrs. Chang, in part because she speaks very little English. Her son and daughter-in-law usually serve as interpreters for communications with the staff, but there are also some Chinese students from the college who visit the nursing home to converse with her.

Mrs. Chang becomes increasingly listless, and spends much of her time sleeping. When blood is discovered in her stools, she is sent to the hospital for diagnostic tests. The tests indicate that she has colon cancer, which has rapidly spread to other parts of her body. An oncologist, Dr. Marilyn Scott, tells her son that the cancer is "too far gone" for chemotherapy or surgery to be viable treatments. Dr. Scott recommends that measures be taken simply to keep her as comfortable as possible until she dies, most likely in just a few months.

Dr. Scott asks Mr. Chang how his mother should be approached with this bad news. Mr. Chang insists that his mother be told absolutely nothing about her condition. He himself does not plan to tell her anything, and he virtually threatens Dr. Scott not to discuss anything with his mother through another interpreter.

> Dr. Scott thinks that Mr. Chang's reaction comes from the initial shock of learning that his mother has a terminal illness. So she asks a physician assistant, Bob Merrill, to approach Mr. Chang again in a few days. However, Mr. Chang reacts to Mr. Merrill in precisely the same way. A week goes by, and Mr. Merrill tries having another conversation with Mr. Chang but he remains adamant in his position.
>
> Dr. Scott thinks that Mrs. Chang could profit from the hospice program available at the nursing home, but her son won't even listen to information about it. Dr. Scott also feels that a do-not-resuscitate order should be discussed with her.
>
> Both Dr. Scott and Mr. Merrill believe strongly that Mr. Chang is being unfair to his mother in not allowing her to be informed of her condition. After all, it's her life and it should be up to her to decide what treatments she does and does not want. Indeed, Dr. Scott has such negative feelings about the way in which Mr. Chang wants to handle the situation and his absolute refusal to agree to "standard medical practice" that she considers withdrawing from the case entirely.

■ ■ ■

Truth-Telling to the Terminally Ill

The case of Mrs. Chang concerns the ethical issue of telling the truth about a terminal condition to a patient. Both the physician and physician assistant involved in her care are concerned that she does not know her diagnosis and hence is unable to make her own decisions about the type and extent of treatment to receive as her life draws to a close. These concerns on the part of health care providers reflect two principles of American health care ethics: truth-telling to the terminally ill and patient autonomy.

Within American health care a distinct change in attitude has taken place concerning truth-telling to the terminally ill. Prior to 1960, the predominant practice was to withhold information from the patient, for fear that frank truth would frighten or harm her. (2) Studies indicate that, in 1960, about 90 percent of cancer physicians favored nondisclosure of the diagnosis. But twenty years later, 90 percent favored disclosure of the diagnostic information to patients. (2) In fact, the *Ethical and Religious Directives for Catholic Health Care Services* in the United States make truth-telling to the terminally ill a matter of policy:

> Persons in danger of death should be provided with whatever information is necessary to help them understand their condition and have the opportunity to discuss their condition with their family members and care providers. They should be offered the appropriate medical information that would make it possible to address the morally legitimate choices available to them. (3)

Various concerns have been expressed about a policy of telling the truth to patients who are terminally ill. For one thing, medical diagnoses and prognoses are never 100 percent certain. We can all think of cases in which someone was expected to die but unexpectedly recovered. So why cause a patient distress unnecessarily? Others have questioned the ability of patients who are debilitated by a serious illness to understand the information given to them, and whether patients in fact want bad news communicated to them. Further, there is concern that announcement of a terminal illness may harm the patient by causing fright or depression, by causing her to cease to struggle against the disease, or even by prompting a cardiac arrest or suicide. (4)

On the other hand, it has been argued that patients often intuitively have a sense of their condition. As Kübler-Ross indicates from her studies with the dying: "When we asked our patients how they had been told, we learned that all the patients know about their terminal illness anyway, whether they were explicitly told or not. . . . " (5) Indeed, patients can be relieved when the issue of their terminal condition is brought out into the open. Proponents of truth-telling also call attention to studies that indicate that a large majority of persons say they would like to be told of the diagnosis of a serious illness. (4) And it is pointed out that a policy of truth-telling in the case of terminal illness is not equivalent to blurting out medical information coldly. Such a policy can and should be accompanied by "finesse, feeling, warmth, empathy, etc., with regard to how much?–when?–how? . . . "(6)

Finally, while concern has been expressed about possible harmful effects on patients of knowing about terminal illness, it is argued that the withholding of information can also have negative consequences:

> . . . we are also becoming increasingly aware of all that can befall patients in the course of their illness when information is denied or distorted. Lies place them in a position where they no longer participate in choices concerning their own health, including the choice of whether to be a "patient" in the first place. A terminally ill person who is not informed that his illness is incurable and that he is near death cannot make decisions about the end of his life; about whether or not to enter a hospital,

or to have surgery; where and with whom to spend his last days; how to put his affairs in order—these most personal choices cannot be made if he is kept in the dark, or given contradictory hints and clues. (4)

Positively stated, truth-telling to terminally ill patients may allow them to participate in decisions about their medical treatment, to make more satisfying use of the time remaining to them, and to make preparations for death. And this is where there is a connection between truth-telling to the terminally ill and patient autonomy. It is argued that patients should be told the truth about their terminal condition precisely so that they themselves can make choices about and direct what happens at the end of their lives.

To someone imbued with the principles of truth-telling and autonomy (as were the physician and physician assistant involved in the care of Mrs. Chang), it might appear that Mrs. Chang's family is not acting in her best interests. A conflict arises in the case of Mrs. Chang precisely because her family is from a culture which brings a different set of beliefs and values to bear in caring for the terminally ill. Many Chinese believe that a person is entitled to be treated as a child when ill, deserving protection. To tell someone that he or she is dying is considered to be not only rude but dangerous, like casting a death curse upon the person which will make the person despair and die even sooner. Thus discussions of code status or the possibility of hospice care are precluded. Further, it is believed that truth telling about a terminal illness signifies the withdrawal of hope, indicating to patients that their health care providers have given up on them and that they might as well "give up" too. While a family may be fully aware of the grave diagnosis, cultural expectations are that they will not acknowledge or discuss it openly. (7)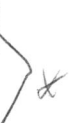

To this Chinese family, telling Mrs. Chang the truth about her terminal illness is a callous act because it is seen as signifying the loss of all hope. Such truth-telling is considered rude and dangerous. Further, an important value to this family is protecting the patient from harm. This value is put into practice by withholding the truth and refraining from any discussions about her impending death. This is a very different mindset from current Western health care practice in which truth telling is seen positively as something that enables the patient to have some control over the end of her life.

How can health care workers identify when a conflict situation with a patient and her family is due to cultural differences? They can try to learn as much as possible about the cultural beliefs and practices of ethnic groups with whom they have contact. (8) To do this, they might "identify one or two individuals from the patient's family or community who are willing to act as cultural informants." (8) Or they might "consult with other health care practitioners from the same ethnic group as the patient." (8) Or again, they might call on the resources of local colleges and universities. (8)

How can health care workers *resolve conflicts* due to cultural differences? In such cases health care workers need to be flexible; they need to show respect for beliefs and practices different than their own; and they need to be willing to compromise. (8) For example, in the case of Mrs. Chang and her family, an accommodation might be achieved between American and Chinese values by her health care providers asking Mrs. Chang if she has any questions about her condition or treatment, and by assuring her family that she will not be told any more than she wishes to know. (8) Ethically, these accommodations to persons of different cultures respect their right to self-determination and autonomy. (8)

Further Examples of Cultural Diversity

Autonomy is a prominent value in contemporary American health care ethics. In the context of end-of-life decision making, the emphasis on autonomy has been described in this way:

> Traditionally, bioethics theory and practice have relied heavily on the Western philosophical principle of respect for persons to justify a model of end-of-life decision making that is focused on the rights and wishes of the individual patient. An important goal of bioethics innovation—such as advance care directives and open disclosure of prognosis—is to promote control of medical decision making at the end of life by an autonomous, fully informed patient.
>
> In the United States, the "ideal" patient is a self-governing individual who is future oriented and willing to engage in frank discussions about difficult medical topics, including planning for his or her own death. (9)

However, "some have argued that this preoccupation with individual rights to the exclusion of other values," such as family integrity and the responsibility of health care professionals, "may reflect a cultural bias on the part of the Western medical and bioethics communities." (10) It has been suggested that "the notion of an informed active decision maker may not be a universally held ideal of the good patient but rather, a very specific set of values based on a particular Western philosophical tradition." (9)

For example, Latinos tend to be group-oriented and family-oriented rather than individualistic. (11) For this reason, health issues are dealt with at the family level. (11)

> . . . giving consent for a diagnostic or surgical procedure is a family affair for most Latinos. Before making a final decision, adults often insist on holding family meetings to seek the advice and opinions of other adult family members, usually brothers, sisters, and even *comadres* ("co-mothers," closest female friends) and *compadres* (male equivalent of comadres). . . . Adult family members are generally responsible for giving consent to carry out a procedure for a spouse, a child, or an elderly person. . . .
>
> Adult children are traditionally responsible for elderly adults, who tend to voluntarily abdicate responsibility for their own health care and well-being. An elderly Latino or Latina very rarely makes major decisions regarding health issues. If consent is requested for a diagnostic or surgical procedure, elderly Latinos will often tell you that the decision is in the hands of their family. Often, brothers and sisters, children, and even grandchildren convene at an urgent family meeting to discuss the issue, and adults take a vote. If one relative lives out of town or in another country, the meeting (and therefore the procedure) may be postponed for a later date to await the arrival of that person. (11)

It has also been noted that "in many Asian societies, ideas about 'selfhood' vary from the western ideal of an autonomous individual" so that a "sociocentric or relational sense of self often leads to decision-making styles at odds with western bioethics ideals." (12)

Another area of cross-cultural difference is pain management. American palliative care specialists emphasize controlling a patient's pain, even to the point of putting patients into a state of diminished consciousness or permanent unconsciousness until death naturally occurs. (See chapter 10.) On the other hand, "mindfulness and mental clarity are important values for Buddhists," as evidenced by the importance placed on meditation. (13) Buddhism emphasizes "the importance of death with an unclouded mind wherever possible." (13) Hence some Buddhists may be "unwilling to take pain-relieving drugs or strong sedatives, and even those who are not in a terminal condition might prefer to remain as alert as possible, rather than take analgesics that would impair their mental or sensory capacities." (13)

Or again, it is commonplace in the United States to have individuals sign a written consent form for a variety of diagnostic tests and medical procedures. However, an Arab who has verbally agreed to a test or procedure may become irate when subsequently asked to sign a written consent form and may refuse to do so. (1) This is because Arabs regard a verbal agreement as "binding and equal to their written agreement." (1) To press them further for a written agreement "only suggests mistrust of their verbal contract" and challenges their personal honor. (1)

What does this cultural diversity mean for ethics and the validity of ethical judgments and practices? Can we ever say for sure that anything is ethically right or wrong?

Ethical Relativism vs. Ethical Objectivism

Multiculturalism in health care raises the question of *ethical objectivism* versus *ethical relativism*. Ethical objectivists maintain that there are some basic ethical standards and values that hold for everyone everywhere. An ethical relativist, on the other hand, denies this and maintains that what is right and wrong varies among different cultures and groups. So, for example, an ethical relativist might maintain that polygamy (the practice of having more than one wife at the same time) is ethically wrong in one country but ethically permissible in another. The ethical relativist does *not* maintain merely that people in the two countries may *think* polygamy is wrong (or right), but that polygamy is *in fact* wrong in one country but right in another. (See chapter 1.)

That different cultural groups consider different things to be ethically right and wrong is often presented as evidence in favor of ethical relativism. For example, Americans favor telling the complete and absolute truth about terminal illness to a patient, whereas (as we have seen) this is considered the wrong thing to do by Chinese people. But does this really mean there are no shared ethical principles among all human beings?

Those favoring ethical objectivism argue that different cultures and groups may share the same basic ethical principles and values but may put these principles and values into practice in different ways because of different circumstances or a different set of factual beliefs. (See chapter 1.) For example, in the case of an Arab agreeing to a medical test or procedure, the basic point of giving consent is really not at issue; the question concerns the way giving consent is practiced. Americans emphasize written consent whereas Arabs place a high value on verbal consent. In the case of Mrs. Chang, we learn that Chinese place a high priority on protecting patients from harm. American health care ethicists adhere to the principle of nonmaleficence, recognizing an obligation of health care workers to prevent harm from coming to patients. (See chapter 1.) The same basic value is held in the two cultures, and the dispute arises over the consequences believed to follow from truth-telling in the case of terminal illness. Chinese see truth-telling as harming the patient by causing her to lose hope and bringing on an earlier death. Americans, on the other hand, have questioned whether these bad effects really come about for most patients and see harm to the patient coming from withholding the truth about terminal illness. If Chinese and Americans could be brought to agree factually on the consequences of truth-telling in the case of terminal illness, they might well agree ethically on whether this should be done.

CHAPTER SUMMARY

Key Terms and Concepts

principle of patient autonomy: self-determination; the right of a patient to make the final decision in matters pertaining to his or her own life and health care.
principle of nonmaleficence: the ethical duty not to inflict harm on others.
ethical objectivism: the position that there are some basic ethical principles that hold for everyone everywhere.
ethical relativism: the position that what is in fact right and wrong varies among different cultures and societies.

Key Points

- Telling a terminally ill patient the truth about her condition is now standard practice in American health care. This is done to allow a patient to participate in decisions about medical treatments, to make more satisfying use of the time remaining to her, and to make appropriate preparations for death. In other words, truth-telling is supposed to enable a patient to better direct and control what happens at the end of her life, and thus follows from the ethical principle of patient autonomy.
- Not all cultures and societies favor telling the truth to a patient who is terminally ill because they regard it as harming the patient.
- American culture emphasizes individual autonomy in health care decision making, whereas other cultures favor a family model of decision making.
- American palliative care practices emphasize controlling pain, even at the cost of putting the patient into a state of diminished consciousness or permanent unconsciousness until death occurs. However, a person from another cultural tradition may value mental lucidity over pain control.
- American health care has adopted a procedure of requiring written consent from the patient or his proxy. Other cultures may not have the same

emphasis and, for example, may attach more importance to verbal assent than does American culture.
- When health care providers are involved in a conflict situation with a patient and/or his family due to cultural differences, they should try to learn about the beliefs and practices of the patient and his family, be flexible, and seek courses of action that can accommodate the cultural beliefs and practices of the patient and his family.
- The fact that beliefs and practices may differ among various cultures and societies does *not* necessarily mean that human beings cannot agree on what is ethically right and wrong and have no shared ethical principles and values. Various cultures and societies may share basic ethical values and principles, but put them into practice in different ways because of different circumstances or factual beliefs.

FOR FURTHER DISCUSSION

1. What ethnic and racial groups are present in your geographical area? How much do you know about their beliefs and practices regarding the provision of health care? Where or from whom can you find out more information?
2. Reflect on your own cultural background and how your extended family approaches health care. Do you see any differences from what is considered "standard practice" in American health care?
3. You are working with Pedro Garcia to help him stop smoking. In order to motivate him, you repeatedly tell him about the harmful effects smoking will have on his own health. However, he is not responding to these warnings. Given that Latinos tend to be group-oriented and family-oriented rather than individualistic, would another kind of message be more effective in motivating him to stop smoking? (11)
4. Do you see any value in a family model of health care decision making in contrast to individual autonomy? Any drawbacks?

References

1. Afaf Ibrahim Meleis & Albert R. Jonsen, "Ethical Crises and Cultural Differences," *The Western Journal of Medicine* 138/6 (June 1983): 889-93.

2. Howard Brody, "The Physician/Patient Relationship" in Robert M. Veatch (ed.), *Medical Ethics* (Boston: Jones and Bartlett, 1989).
3. United States Conference of Catholic Bishops, *Ethical and Religious Directives for Catholic Health Care Services* (2001), no. 55. http://www.usccb.org. Accessed April 2009.
4. Sissela Bok, "Lies to the Sick and Dying" in *Lying: Moral Choice in Public and Private Life* (New York: Pantheon, 1978).
5. Elisabeth Kübler-Ross, *On Death and Dying* (New York: Macmillan, 1969).
6. Orville N. Griese, *Catholic Identity in Health Care: Principles and Practice* (Braintree: MA: Pope John Center, 1987).
7. Jessica H. Muller & Brian Desmond, "Ethical Dilemmas in a Cross-cultural Context A Chinese Example," *The Western Journal of Medicine* 157/3 (September 1992): 323-27.
8. Robert D. Orr, Patricia A. Marshall & Jamie Osborn, "Cross-cultural Considerations in Clinical Ethics Consultations," *Archives of Family Medicine* 4 (February 1995): 159-64.
9. Patricia A. Marshall, Barbara A. Koenig, Donelle M. Barnes, and Anne J. Davis, "Multiculturalism, Bioethics, and End-of-Life Care: Case Narratives of Latino Cancer Patients," in John F. Monagle and David C. Thomasma (eds.), *Health Care Ethics: Critical Issues for the 21st Century* (Gaithersburg, MD: Aspen, 1998).
10. Leslie J. Blackhall, Sheila T. Murphy, Gelya Frank, Vicki Michel, and Stanley Azen, "Ethnicity and Attitudes Toward Patient Autonomy," *Journal of the American Medical Association* 274/10 (Sept. 13, 1995): 820-25.
11. Nilda Chong, *The Latino Patient A Cultural Guide for Health Care Providers* (Yarmouth, Maine: Intercultural Press, 2002).
12. Barbara A. Koenig and Jan Gates-Williams, "Understanding Cultural Difference in Caring for Dying Patients," *Western Journal of Medicine* 163/3 (Sept. 1995): 244-49.
13. Damien Keown, "End of Life: the Buddhist view," *The Lancet* 366 (Sept. 10, 2005): 952-55.

Part Four
Special Topics

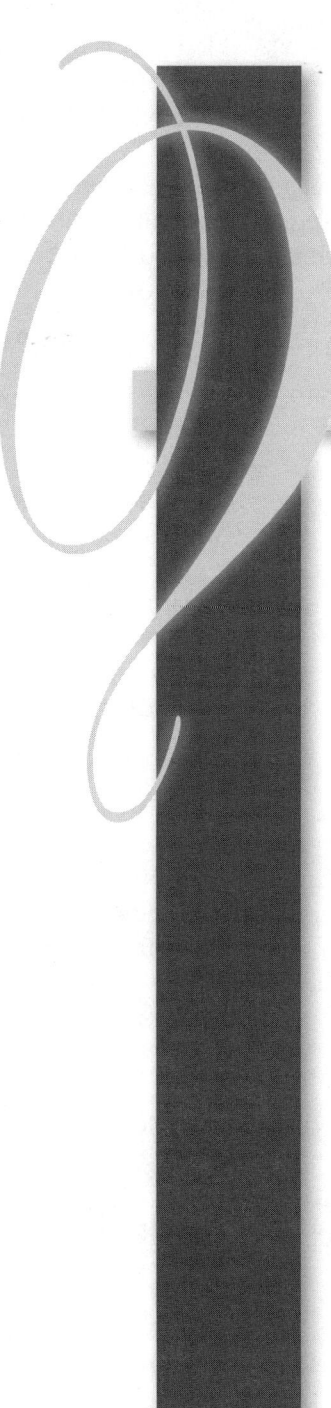

Chapter 15

Research and Experimentation Involving Human Subjects

The Nuremberg trials following World War II brought to light medical research and experimentation conducted by the Nazis that were abusive of human subjects. These abuses were prevalent in the concentration camps. At Dachau, for example, "healthy inmates were injected with extracts from the mucous glands of mosquitoes to produce malaria" and then various drugs were "used to determine their relative effectiveness." (1) At Buchenwald, "various kinds of poisons were secretly administered to a number of inmates to test their efficacy." (1) At Ravensbrück, people were deliberately cut and their wounds infected with bacteria in order to test the efficacy of the drug sulfanilamide. (1)

Unfortunately, medical experiments abusive of human beings were not limited to Nazi Germany. Questionable research projects have also been conducted within the United States. A prime example is the Tuskegee Syphilis Study conducted under the auspices of the U.S. Department of Public Health:

> From 1932 to 1970, a large but undetermined number of black males suffering from the later stages of syphilis were examined at regular intervals to determine the course their disease was taking. The men in the study were poor and uneducated . . . they were given either no treatment or inadequate treatment, and at least forty of them died as a result of factors connected with their disease. . . . It was known when the study began that those with untreated syphilis have a higher death rate than those whose condition is treated, and although the study was started before the advent of penicillin (which is highly effective against syphilis), other drugs were available but were not used in ways to produce the best results. When penicillin became generally available, it still was not used. (1)

This is not an isolated incident. From the 1940s to the 1960s, chemical testing involving mescaline and LSD was conducted by the American military and intelligence agencies. Experiments took place without the knowledge of the subjects and sometimes resulted in death. (2) Also controversial were the Willowbrook hepatitis experiments, which involved mentally challenged children in a state institution as research subjects. (1)

Such abusive practices have led to the formulation of *codes of research ethics* such as the *Nuremberg Code* (3), the *Declaration of Helsinki* of the World Medical Association (4), and the Belmont Report (5). Within the United States, health care facilities and research institutes have established institutional review boards (IRBs) to review and approve proposed research projects as a condition for receiving funding from the U.S. Department of Health and Human Services. (2)

In this chapter you will learn about:

- general norms and specific criteria used to evaluate proposed research projects;
- ethical principles underlying these norms and criteria;
- challenges in obtaining informed consent from potential research subjects;
- restrictions on proxy consent for participation in research and experimentation.

Case Study

Marilyn Stewart provides occupational therapy services at Sun Valley Care Center. When she makes her visit this week, the administrator calls Marilyn into his office. He tells her that researchers at the state university medical school are conducting a study of a new blood pressure medication using the residents of Sun Valley. This new medication is expected to have fewer of the unpleasant side effects many older persons experience with the currently standard medications. However, the administrator points out that "you can never be sure exactly what to expect with medication that is still being tested." He asks Marilyn to watch for unusual symptoms or behavior on the part of residents—which may be a function of the medication—and to alert a nurse on duty about it.

Marilyn notices that the administrator seems quite proud that his facility was chosen by researchers at the state university's medical school to participate in this study. However, she wonders how much the residents understand about the research project in which they are the experimental subjects. Some of the residents are hard of hearing and have poor eyesight. Some suffer from memory loss. Some suffer from dementia, in varying degrees. What kind of explanation of the research study was given to the residents? And how much of the explanation did they understand? Who made the decision that the residents should participate in this research project? Marilyn wonders if the residents of whom she has grown so fond are simply being used as "guinea pigs."

■ ■ ■

Norms and Criteria for Evaluating Proposed Research Projects

Before this new blood pressure medication could be administered to the residents of Sun Valley Care Center, the researchers would have been required to submit a proposal to the Institutional Review Board (IRB) at the university's medical school to conduct this study. The members of the IRB would review their research protocol to ensure proper protection for the human subjects to be used in the research project. In their review, the members of the IRB might use something like the following worksheet.

IRB WORKSHEET

... research will be founded on the four basic principles for human conduct: beneficence (doing good), nonmaleficence (not harming), respecting persons and justice. The proposal is reviewed using six ethical norms for research involving human subjects founded on these principles. The criteria listed are conditions each of which must be satisfied for a project to be ethically legitimate ...

1. Good research design
   1.1 Based on a thorough knowledge of the scientific literature.
   1.2 Designed and based on results of experimentation at the pre-human level, if available.
   1.3 Conforms to generally accepted scientific principles.
   1.4 Expected to yield fruitful results for the good of society, unprocurable by other methods or means of study.
   1.5 Conducted so as to avoid all unnecessary physical and mental suffering and injury.
   1.6 Importance of the objective is in proportion to the inherent risk to the subject.
   1.7 Confidentiality: Every precaution is taken to respect the privacy of the subject and to minimize the impact of the study on the subject's physical and mental integrity and on the personality of the subject. In publication of the results, the doctor is obliged to preserve the accuracy of the results.
2. Balance of harm and benefit
   2.1 Degree of risk to be taken does not exceed that determined by the humanitarian importance of the problem to be solved by the experiment.
   2.2 Preceded by careful assessment of predictable risks in comparison with foreseeable benefits to the subject or to others.
   2.3 Concern for the interests of the subject always prevails over the interest of science and society.
3. Competence of the investigator(s)
   3.1 Investigator (or investigative team) has adequate training and skill to accomplish the purposes of the research.
   3.2 Supervision by a clinically competent medical person.

3.3 A high degree of professionalism with evidence of responsibility for the human subject.

4. Informed consent
   4.1 Voluntary consent of the human subject is absolutely essential.
   4.2 Person involved has legal capacity to give consent (OR if the person is legally incompetent, guardian consents; OR if a minor, responsible relative consent in addition to minor consent).
   4.3 Person or proxy acknowledges sufficient knowledge and comprehension of the elements of the research project (aims, methods, anticipated benefits and potential hazards of the study and the discomfort it may entail).
   4.4 Free power of choice: The prospective subject or proxy is in no way highly dependent upon those who would be seeking consent.
   4.5 Person or proxy maintains the right to withdraw at any time without prejudice.
   4.6 Person or proxy will be informed that results of the study will be made available to him/her upon request.
   4.7 In instances of nontherapeutic experimentation, the proxy can give his consent only if the experiment entails no significant risk to the person's well-being. Moreover, the greater the person's incompetence and vulnerability, the greater the reasons must be to perform any medical experimentation, especially nontherapeutic.

5. Equitable selection of subjects
   5.1 Patient population: Distribution of subjects is randomized and not solely those who are less advantaged.
   5.2 Protection of the vulnerable: no use of institutionalized subjects (prisoners) or persons with limited capacities to consent.
   5.3 Subjects should be volunteers.
   5.4 Subjects should be protected from arbitrary turn down without criteria.

6. Compensation for research-related injury
   6.1 Provision exists to discontinue research that is determined to likely result in injury, disability or death to the experimental subject.
   6.2 Subjects who suffer physical, psychological or social injury in the course of research shall be compensated 1) if the injury is primarily caused by such research and 2) if the injury exceeds that reasonably associated with such illness from which the subject may be suffering, as well as with treatment usually associated with such illness at the time the subject began participating in the research. (6)

From an ethical point of view, this IRB Worksheet is noteworthy in starting out with four fundamental ethical principles—beneficence, nonmaleficence, respecting persons, and justice (cf. principalism in chapter 1)—and deriving from them six more specific norms for evaluating proposed research projects, namely, good research design, balance of harm and benefit, competence of the investigators, informed consent, equitable selection of subjects, and compensation for research-related injury. Exactly how do the six norms follow from the four fundamental principles?

The norms of good research design and competence of the investigator(s) are related to the principle of beneficence. For "without a competent investigator (or investigative team) and good research design, there will be no benefits forthcoming from the study." (7) These two norms are also related to the principle of nonmaleficence. This is so because "competent investigators and good research design also protect subjects from harm." (7) Further, "the requirements that the investigator(s) be competent and the research well designed serve to ensure that people's time is not wasted and that their desire to participate in a meaningful activity is not frustrated." (7) These two norms also uphold the principle of respect for persons. (7)

The norm of balancing harm and benefit is derived from both the principle of beneficence (doing good) and the principle of nonmaleficence (avoiding harm).

The principle of respecting persons comes from the philosopher Immanuel Kant and "requires that persons not be used merely as a means to another's end." (7) The norm of informed consent upholds this principle by ensuring that research subjects "are not 'used' by another without their knowledge and consent." (7)

The principle of justice requires fairness in the distribution of benefits and of burdens. Justice is the foundation for the norm requiring an equitable selection of subjects. The "burdens" of research activity are the risks involved in experimentation, and it would be unfair to make the less advantaged and the vulnerable in society take all the risks. Obviously, the principle of justice also serves as the foundation for the norm concerning compensation for research-related injury.

How does the blood pressure medication research project at Sun Valley Care Center stand up against these norms (and the more specific criteria for implementing them)? While we do not have enough detail about this research project to comment on each of the specific criteria listed in the IRB Worksheet, there are several points which stand out and deserve comment.

Any research project involves a balancing of benefits and risks for the human subjects participating in it (see IRB Worksheet 2.2). This is clearly illustrated in the case of Sun Valley Care Center. The occupational therapist Marilyn Stewart is cautioned by Sun Valley's administrator to watch for unusual symptoms or behavior in residents that may be caused by the medication being tested. These possible undesirable effects constitute the risks of this particular research study. These risks are counterbalanced by the expected benefits of the new medication, namely, that the residents will experience fewer of the unpleasant side effects of the currently standard blood pressure medications.

There has been a problem with persons living in an institutional setting, such as a long-term care facility, being used as research subjects as a matter of convenience:

> Historically, nursing home patients were used as research participants disproportionately to their representation in the population, as were prisoners and other institutionalized groups, primarily for the convenience of the investigator. If the researcher can get all the subjects in one place, it is much easier to collect samples, do interviews, or conduct follow-up of the research. For example, it was much easier to get the consent of prisoners to participate by giving trivial amounts of money (or in some cases cartons of cigarettes) than it would have been to obtain consent from people in the community who have greater freedom. The studies were not particularly or especially relevant to problems of prisoners or problems of nursing home patients and therefore it was thought that this kind of selection bias was inequitable. (8)

Since medical research benefits society as a whole, there should, as a matter of justice, be an "equitable distribution of the burdens of participation in research." (8) This entails that "populations not be selected simply for the convenience of the investigator, but that they be selected for true representativeness related to the sample selection needs of the study." (8) Thus one criterion of legitimate research and experimentation is that subjects be selected equitably. No one group of persons should be used exclusively since this involves the possibility of exploiting certain groups in society, especially those who are less advantaged (see IRB Worksheet 5.1).

As far as we know, the new blood pressure medication is being tested *only* at Sun Valley Care Center. If, for example, Sun Valley were a county facility for indigent elderly persons (versus a nursing home where residents pay their own expenses), we would have good reason to worry that the research project was "using" poor people. However, we have no reason to think that Sun Valley is this type of facility. At the same time, we may worry that *only* the residents of Sun Valley are subjects in the research study. Are they being taken advantage of because they are in a nursing home? Why does the research study not include some elderly persons still living at home? (9)

Occupational therapist Marilyn Stewart notes a concern about the level of understanding the residents have of the project in which they are participating and the related issue of consent to participation. This is an issue which deserves extended examination.

Free and Informed Consent

A prominent principle in contemporary health care ethics is *patient autonomy*. Autonomy refers to self-determination. The principle of patient autonomy affirms the right of a patient to make the final decision in matters pertaining to his or her own life, including his or her health care. The requirement to obtain the free and informed consent of an individual to participate in research and experimentation (see IRB Worksheet 4.1-4.4) is often grounded in patient autonomy as well as in the principle of respect for persons. (5)

Federal regulations specify that the following information be provided to a potential research subject as basic elements of informed consent:

- A statement that the study involves research, an explanation of the purposes of the research and the expected duration of the subject's participation, a description of the procedures to be followed, and identification of any procedures which are experimental;
- A description of any reasonably foreseeable risks or discomforts to the subject;
- A description of any benefits to the subject or to others which may reasonably be expected from the research;
- A disclosure of appropriate alternative procedures or courses of treatment, if any, that might be advantageous to the subject;
- A statement describing the extent, if any, to which confidentiality of records identifying the subject will be maintained;
- For research involving more than minimal risk, an explanation as to whether any compensation and an explanation as to whether any medical treatments are available if injury occurs and, if so, what they consist of, or where further information may be obtained;
- An explanation of whom to contact for answers to pertinent questions about the research and research subjects' rights, and whom to contact in the event of a research-related injury to the subject; and

- A statement that participation is voluntary, refusal to participate will involve no penalty or loss of benefits to which the subject is otherwise entitled, and the subject may discontinue participation at any time without penalty or loss of benefits to which the subject is otherwise entitled. (10)

It is standard practice that a potential research subject (or his proxy) sign a written consent form to participate in the research project.

There are various challenges to obtaining truly free and informed consent from patients to participate in research projects. One challenge to "informed" consent is using language that is understandable to the potential research subjects in the consent forms that they must sign. Many consent forms "require the potential volunteer to 'synthesize information from complex or lengthy passages'. . . or to 'make high-level inferences or use specialized background knowledge' about medicine . . .". (11) Based on the results of the National Adult Literacy Survey (1993), it is estimated that only 3 percent to 20 percent of American adults have the reading skills needed to understand current research consent forms. (11) Moreover, the survey indicated that people with a chronic illness, disability, or impairment have even lower levels of literacy skills than the total sample. (11) This finding is especially relevant to the case involving the residents of Sun Valley Care Center in evaluating their ability to give informed consent to participation in the blood pressure medication research project.

As an illustration of the problem about using understandable language, consider the following excerpt from a consent form for trial of a new drug (IND):

> You will initially receive 50 milligrams (mg) of [IND] per kilogram (kg) of your body weight, followed by 25 mg/kg every 6 hours for 4 days, followed by 12.5 mg/kg every 6 hours for 6 days. (11)

This statement is not likely to give any clear information about dosage levels to someone who is not a health care worker. Consider a possible revision of it:

> The first dose will start right away. We will give bigger doses in the first 4 days, and smaller doses the last 6 days. Those are the same doses used for many years to treat other diseases. (11)

Not only is the language here much simpler and less technical, but the revision has the advantage of addressing a question potential research subjects will probably have. Few subjects are likely to want to know exactly how many milligrams of an experimental drug they will receive. They are more likely to want to know whether the dosage level is itself part of the experiment or if the same dose was found effective in previous research. The revision answers this question in a clear and straightforward way. (11)

Other problems with obtaining truly informed consent concern the amount and detail of the information that is communicated. Studies indicate that the longer the consent form, the smaller the number of people that read the form in its entirety. This results in less, rather than more information being conveyed. (11) Further, extensive detail "usually enhances the subject's confusion." (12) Studies again indicate that the more elaborate the material presented to potential research subjects, the less they understand. (12) Indeed, an investigator "conceivably could exploit his authority and knowledge and extract 'informed consent' by overwhelming the candidate-subject with information." (12) Researchers face the challenge of constructing consent forms that contain all the essential information but still are concise and relatively brief.

The communication process for obtaining a research subject's consent can be enhanced through the use of videotapes or portable flip cards that summarize key points in large print and contain graphics and diagrams. (11) The latter might be especially helpful in working with the residents of Sun Valley Care Center, some of whom have poor eyesight and are hard of hearing. It has also been found that the procedure of "next day consent" improves the communication process. Soliciting consent takes place in a two-stage process, spread over at least twenty-four hours. This gives time for more information to be absorbed by potential research subjects and for discussion with their family members. (11)

A potential subject's consent should be free as well as informed (see IRB Worksheet 4.1, 4.3). As pointed out by the U.S. Department of Health and Human Services, certain categories of potential research subjects "are likely to be vulnerable to coercion or undue influence, such as persons with acute or severe physical or mental illness, or persons who are economically or educationally disadvantaged." (13) The pressures which operate can be subtle ones. Consider, for example, the situation of patients in hospitals:

> Patients are psychologically predisposed to act in ways that please physicians. Not only do physicians possess a social role that makes them figures of authority, but an ill person feels very dependent on those who may possess the power to make him well. Thus, he will be inclined to go along with any suggestion or recommendation made by a physician. The ordinary patient, like the inmate in an institution, needs protection from the social and psychological pressures that are exerted by circumstances. Otherwise, the voluntariness of consent will be compromised. . . . (1)

Long-term care facilities (like Sun Valley Care Center in our case) and mental hospitals are *total institutions* within which "all aspects of a person's life are connected with the social structure." (1) In turn, there can be social forces operating to encourage and pressure a resident or patient to do what is expected of him or her. (1) These subtle forms of pressure are undoubtedly the reason behind stipulation 4.3 in the IRB Worksheet: "The prospective subject or proxy is in no way highly dependent upon those who would be seeking consent."

Proxy Consent for Participation in Research and Experimentation

In our case, occupational therapist Marilyn Stewart notes that some of the residents of Sun Valley Care Center who are subjects in the blood pressure medication experiment are suffering from dementia, in varying degrees. Some of them may not have the capacity themselves to give free and informed consent to participate in the research project. Indeed, Marilyn raises the question of who made the decision about the residents participating in it.

In the case of mentally incapacitated adults and minors, proxy consent is recognized as legitimate. This is indicated in the IRB Worksheet: "Person involved has legal capacity to give consent (OR if person is legally incompetent, guardian consent; OR if a minor, responsible relative consent in addition to minor consent)." (4.2) However, some ethicists draw a distinction between *consenting for oneself* and the role of *consenting for another*, placing restrictions on the latter type of consent.

Medical research and experimentation is considered therapeutic if it has the potential to benefit the subjects participating in the project. On the other hand, research and experimentation is classified as nontherapeutic if it is not expected to benefit the subjects themselves but will allow the researchers to gain knowledge which will benefit other patients. Some ethicists hold that proxy decision makers cannot licitly give consent to research and experimentation that is nontherapeutic in character. (1, 14) Their reasoning is that a proxy decision maker has a duty to act in the best interests of the person he represents and for the welfare of that person. (1, 14) Other ethicists take a less restrictive position, allowing for proxy consent to research and experimentation which poses only minimal risk to the subject. (14) Point 4.7 of the IRB Worksheet given above allows for proxy consent for nontherapeutic research and experimentation, with certain qualifications: "In instances of nontherapeutic experimentation, the proxy can give his consent only if the experiment entails no significant risk to the person's well-being. Moreover, the greater the person's incompetence and vulnerability, the greater the reasons must be to perform any medical experimentation, especially nontherapeutic."

These stipulations and restrictions do not pose problems for the research project being carried on at Sun Valley Care Center. The new blood pressure medication being tested is expected to have fewer of the unpleasant side effects many older persons experience with the currently standard medications. If the new medication works as expected, it will clearly be of benefit to those taking it. Thus, this project qualifies as therapeutic research for the residents participating in the project. Even those residents suffering from dementia may be included in the project, with the consent of the appropriate proxy decision maker.

CHAPTER SUMMARY

Key Terms and Concepts

principle of beneficence: the moral duty to act for the benefit and welfare of others.

principle of nonmaleficence: the moral duty not to inflict harm on others.

principle of respecting persons: a principle referring to the views of the philosopher Immanuel Kant, who maintained that we should always treat human persons as having inherent worth and that we act wrongly when we merely "use" people as a means to obtain something else.

principle of justice: a principle concerning fairness in the distribution of benefits, burdens, and resources.

principle of autonomy: self-determination; the right of a patient to make the final decision in matters pertaining to his or her own life and health care.

therapeutic research and experimentation: research and experimentation that has the potential to benefit the subjects participating in it.

nontherapeutic research and experimentation: research and experimentation that is not expected to benefit the subjects participating in it, but will allow researchers to gain knowledge to benefit other patients.

Key Points

- Abuses have occurred in the past with the use of human beings in medical research and experimentation. These abuses have resulted in the formulation of codes of research ethics and the establishment of IRBs (institutional review boards).

- An IRB will review proposed research projects using such norms as good research design, the balance of harm and benefit involved in the project, the competence of the investigator(s), informed consent, whether the subjects of the experiment have been selected equitably, and provision for compensation for research-related injury. These norms follow from the ethical principles of autonomy, beneficence, nonmaleficence, justice and respect for persons. More specific criteria are developed for implementing these general norms.
- The process of obtaining informed consent from a potential research subject involves giving the individual a description of the expected benefits of a research project and its potential discomforts and risks, of alternatives that might be advantageous, and of the procedures to be followed. Subjects must also be informed that they may refuse to participate in the project. Normally all of this information is provided in a written consent form.
- Challenges in obtaining informed consent include presenting information in language that is understandable to potential research subjects, and constructing consent forms that contain all essential information while still being concise and relatively brief.
- Consent to participate in research projects should be free as well as informed. Researchers need to be sensitive to subtle coercive forces that can influence the consent of patients and residents. These coercive forces include the state of dependency of patients and residents on their health care providers and the fact that all aspects of a resident's life in a long-term care facility are connected with the institution's social structure.
- Proxy consent for participation in medical research and experimentation is considered legitimate in the case of minors and mentally incapacitated adults. However, ethicists tend to limit the range of legitimate proxy consent to projects which involve only minimal risk for the participating subject, or sometimes more narrowly to projects which are therapeutic in nature.

FOR FURTHER DISCUSSION

1. Rose Stillman and Michael Bauer are occupational therapists who work at a university medical center. They have both become interested in music therapy. They want to conduct a research project which will consist in playing Gregorian chant to agitated Alzheimer's patients and observing them to determine if the music has a calming effect on their behavior. (15)

    Divide the class into two groups. Let the first group represent the researchers Rose Stillman and Michael Bauer, and let the second group represent an Institutional Review Board (IRB) for the facility at which their research project will be conducted.

The researchers should construct a proposal for their project to submit for IRB approval.

This group will need to develop the details of the projected research project beyond the description given. (HINT: The proposal should include the following information: the purpose of the research project and the researcher's hypothesis; methods and procedures for conducting the research; the number, age range, and gender of participants, and how and where they will be recruited/selected; potential benefits and risks of the project; procedures for informed consent; how the data collected will be handled in terms of confidentiality; the credentials of the researchers.)

The second group should role play a meeting of the IRB to discuss and approve or reject the proposal submitted to them. Does the proposal address and satisfy the various criteria for legitimate experimentation on humans set out in this chapter?

2. When the disease AIDS became prominent, complaints were voiced about the slowness of the U.S. Food and Drug Administration (FDA) in testing and approving drugs which might benefit persons with AIDS. Should patients with life-limiting illnesses have access to any drug they might wish to try, even if research and testing on it have not yet been completed? Should we be guided in these decisions by the ethical principle of autonomy or the ethical principle of nonmaleficence? (16)

3. It is possible to sustain by technological means the vital functions of an individual who has suffered brain death. It has been proposed that such legally dead human beings be sustained specifically for use as subjects in medical research experiments. (17, 18, 19) From an ethical point of view, do you see any problems with doing this?

References

1. "Medical Experimentation and Informed Consent" in Ronald Munson (ed.), *Intervention and Reflection: Basic Issues in Medical Ethics*, 5th ed. (Belmont, CA: Wadsworth, 1996).

2. A.M. Capron, "Human Experimentation" in Robert M. Veatch (ed.), *Medical Ethics* (Boston: Jones & Bartlett, 1989).
3. *Trials of War Criminals before the Nuremberg Military Tribunals under Control Council Law No. 10,* vol. 2 (Washington, D.C.: United States Government Printing Office, 1949).
4. Adopted by the 18th World Medical Assembly, Helsinki, Finland, 1964; revised 1975, 1983, 1989. Reprinted in the *Encyclopedia of Bioethics*, rev. ed. (New York: Macmillan, 1995).
5. National Commission for the Protection of Human Subjects of Biomedical and Behavioral Research, *The Belmont Report Ethical Principles and Guidelines for the protection of human subjects of research* (1979). http://ohsr.od.nih.gov/guidelines/belmont.html. Accessed February 2009.
6. *Research Manual,* Mercy Medical Center, Dubuque, IA (1996).
7. Robert J. Levine & Karen Lebacqz, "Ethical Considerations in Clinical Trials," *Clinical Pharmacology and Therapeutics* 25/5-2 (May 1979).
8. Christine Cassel, "Ethical Issues in the Conduct of Research in Long Term Care," *The Gerontologist* 28 Suppl. (1988): 90-6.
9. Christine Cassel, "Research in Nursing Homes Ethical Issues," *Journal of the American Geriatrics Society* 33/11 (Nov. 1985): 795-99.
10. Code of Federal Regulations, Title 45 Public Welfare; Department of Health and Human Services, Part 46 Protection of Human Subjects, 46.116 General Requirements for Informed Consent. http://www.hhs.gov/ohrp/humansubjects/guidance//45cfr46.htm. Accessed February 2009.
11. William L. Freeman, "Making Research Consent Forms Informative and Understandable: The Experience of the Indian Health Service," *Cambridge Quarterly of Health care Ethics* 3 (1994): 510-21.
12. F.J. Ingelfinger, "Informed (But Uneducated) Consent," *New England Journal of Medicine* 287/9 (August 31, 1972): 465-66.
13. United States Department of Health and Human Services, *Policy for the Protection of Human Research Subjects* 46.111 (7b) in 46 FR 8386, January 26, 1981, 48 FR 9269, March 4, 1983.
14. Benedict M. Ashley, OP & Kevin D. O'Rourke, OP, *Healthcare Ethics: A Theological Analysis,* 3rd ed. (St. Louis: Catholic Health Association, 1989).
15. See, for example. Dr. Alice Cash, *Healing Music Enterprises.* http://www.healingmusic.com/ cvitae.html. Accessed February 2009.

16. "Drug Testing, Autonomy, and Access to Unapproved Drugs" in Ronald Munson (ed.), *Intervention and Reflection: Basic Issues in Medical Ethics,* 5th ed. (Belmont, CA: Wadsworth, 1996).
17. Willard Gaylin, "Harvesting the Dead," *Harpers* 249 (September 1974): 23-26.
18. R. Carson, J. Frias & R. Melker, "Case Study: Research with Brain-Dead Children," *IRB* 3/1 (1981): 5-6.
19. S. Martyn, "Using the Brain Dead for Medical Research," *Utah Law Review* (1986): 1-28.

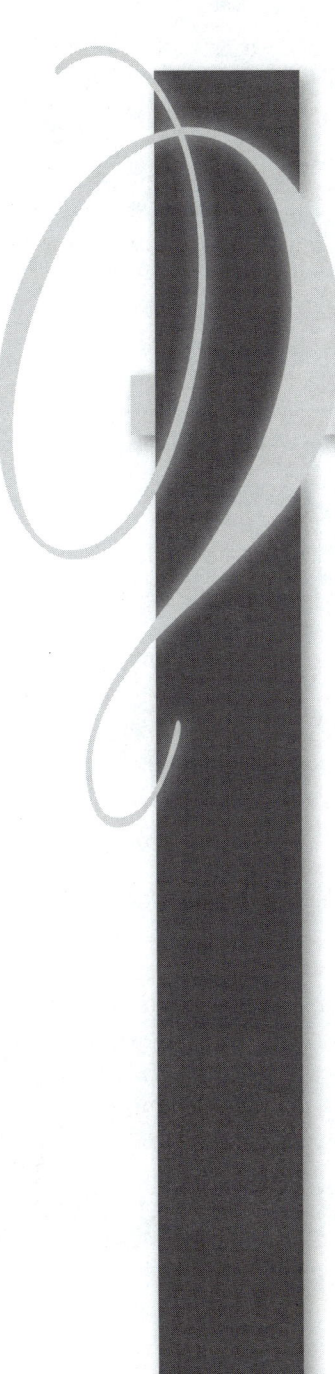

Chapter 16

Stem Cell Research

Some issues in health care ethics, such as confidentiality or forgoing life-sustaining treatments, are perennial ones. Other issues emerge with the advent of new diseases (such as AIDS) or with new developments in scientific and medical research (such as the Human Genome Project). One issue that has become prominent in the twenty-first century is stem cell research.

In this chapter you will learn:

- basic biological information about stem cells;
- ethical questions about deriving stem cells from early embryos;
- ethical concerns surrounding cloning human beings to obtain stem cells.

Case Study

Tim Murphy, 78, was widowed five years ago. Since the death of his wife, he has been using home health care services. His mobility is limited because of arthritis and, as he puts it, a "worn out" hip and knee. Within the last year, the home health care staff visiting him has noticed that he has slowed down considerably. Lately he coughs when he drinks liquids, which makes the staff suspect swallowing problems.

The staff of the home health care service persuades Tim to make an appointment with a neurologist, who diagnoses Tim as in early stage Parkinson's disease. Arrangements are made for Tim to work with a speech therapist about his swallowing problem.

Tim's daughter, Martha, accompanies him to see the speech therapist, Rebecca Smith. Rebecca discusses with Tim and Martha how his diet can be managed to assist him in swallowing. Rebecca also mentions a research project going on at a local university medical center for patients with Parkinson's disease. The research project involves a therapy using stem cells, replacing the dopamine-producing cells in the brains of Parkinson's patients. Rebecca offers to contact the medical center to see if Tim can be enrolled in the project.

Initially, Martha is excited about the availability of a therapy that could help her father and prevent the progress of his Parkinson's disease. Martha has a close friend whose mother suffered from Parkinson's disease for ten years before her death, and she knows how devastating a disease it can be.

At the same time, Martha remembers from her college biology course the controversy that has surrounded the development of therapies from stem cells. Martha has always considered herself to be "pro-life," and she wonders about the ethics of using therapies dependent on stem cells. For this reason, she tells Rebecca Smith that she wants to learn more about these therapies and to consult with her pastor before pursuing the experimental treatment for her father.

■ ■ ■

The Science of Stem Cells: The Basics

The various tissues and organs of the human body consist of specialized cells adapted to perform certain functions; for example, blood cells, heart cells, muscle cells, brain cells. Stem cells are cells that are capable of dividing and renewing themselves for long periods, are unspecialized, and can give rise to specialized cell types. (1)

There are various sources of stem cells. They can be obtained from embryos, adult tissues, umbilical cord blood, and amniotic fluid (with the stem cells lodging in the placenta). (2, 3) They have also been found in women's menstrual blood. (4) It is likewise possible to genetically reprogram adult cells to an embryonic stem cell-like state. These are called induced pluripotent stem cells. (1) Although stem cells can be obtained from fetuses (2), this is not currently an area of emphasis in stem cell research. It is the use of embryonic stem cells that has become a topic of intense ethical debate.

Embryonic stem cells "are derived from embryos that develop from eggs that have been fertilized in vitro—in an in vitro fertilization clinic—and then donated for research purposes with the informed consent of the donors." (1) At the blastocyst stage of development, which occurs around day four or five, the blastocyst has three structures: the trophoblast, an outer ring of cells that will develop into the placenta; the blastocoel, a hollow cavity inside the blastocyst; and the inner cell mass, that will develop into the fetus. Human embryonic stem cells are isolated by transferring the inner cell mass into a laboratory culture dish. Obviously, this destroys the embryo as such. Ultimately, the intent is to coax the stem cells into differentiating into the desired tissue, which would then be placed into the body of the recipient. (1, 5)

However, such transplantation faces the well-known problem of immune rejection because the stem cells derived from the embryos will be genetically different from the recipient's genome. One method for overcoming this problem, which researchers are exploring, is cloning. In a procedure known as somatic cell nuclear transfer (SCNT), the nuclear DNA is removed from an unfertilized ovum and replaced with the nuclear DNA of a somatic cell (a non-reproductive body cell) from the intended recipient of the procedure. The new cell receives a jolt of electricity to begin cell division and growth. When the appropriate stage of embryonic development is reached, the aforementioned procedure for obtaining stem cells will be used. This procedure is known as "therapeutic cloning" to distinguish it from "reproductive cloning," the potential use of cloning to produce a live born child. (2, 6) However, SCNT will not give a perfect genetic match "because mitochondrial genes would come from the donor egg cell," and thus "there is a potential for exposure of foreign mitochondrial proteins that could cause tissue rejection." (2) Hence "patients may still require taking antirejection medications though the dosage may be lower." (2)

First and foremost, there is intense interest in stem cell research because of therapies that could be developed. Stem cells could generate cells and tissues to treat a variety of diseases, such as Parkinson's, Alzheimer's, spinal cord injury, stroke, burns, heart disease, diabetes, and arthritis. (1) Further, the need for transplantable tissues and organs exceeds the available supply, and tissues and organs grown from stem cells might help meet this need. (1) Studies of human embryonic stem cells are expected to yield information about the events that occur during human development, especially cell differentiation to form tissues and organs. This, in turn, could provide insight into serious medical conditions such as cancer and birth defects, which are due to abnormal cell division and differentiation. (1) Finally, stem cells could be used to produce differentiated cells for testing new drugs. (1)

Stem cell research is a rapidly developing area of scientific research. For this reason, supplementary resources should be consulted to become informed about the latest work and advances in stem cell research.

The Ethics of Stem Cell Research

Stem cell research is often presented in a black and white fashion: one is either for it or against it. From an ethical point of view, distinctions must be made among different types of stem cell research. Research utilizing stem cells derived from sources other than embryos (or aborted fetuses) has not been controversial ethically (7, 8), although such research must be conducted in accord with accepted standards for medical research and experimentation on humans. (See chapter 15.) What is ethically controversial, in terms of the current practice of stem cell research, is embryonic stem cell research and therapeutic cloning.

Obtaining stem cells from embryos involves the destruction of early stage embryos. Thus one's judgment about the ethical permissibility of embryonic stem cell research is dependent on one's judgment whether the early stage embryo constitutes a human being with a right to life. (See the discussion of this issue in chapter 3.)

Even if one considers the early stage embryo to be a human being, some argue that it is still permissible to use spare frozen embryos from fertility clinics in stem cell research. The process of in vitro fertilization typically involves retrieving and fertilizing a number of ova. However, not all the embryos created are transferred to a woman's body at a given time to try to achieve a pregnancy; this is done to prevent multifetal pregnancies. Remaining embryos may be frozen for later use. However, frozen embryos may become "spare" if a couple achieves the child they want and does not want to keep any remaining frozen embryos for future attempts at having children. Or sometimes the IVF procedure simply does not work to achieve a pregnancy and a discouraged couple gives up trying, although some frozen embryos they have created remain. Such spare frozen embryos may simply be destroyed, or they are sometimes offered to infertile couples for adoption. (9) Thus the argument is made that, if spare frozen embryos are destined to be destroyed anyway, they ought to be donated for research (such as stem cell research) which will benefit other persons therapeutically. (7)

One ethicist has formalized this line of argument by using a maxim he denominates the "nothing-is-lost" principle and extending it from certain kinds of conflict cases to the case of spare frozen embryos destined to be destroyed (10):

> The nothing-is-lost principle, as understood by Outka, is intended to permit the use of lethal force in cases of conflict. In Outka's formulation, "One may directly kill when two conditions obtain: (a) the innocent will die in any case; and (b) other innocent life will be saved." In the case of embryos, Outka wishes to extend the principle in the following way: One may directly kill if "(a) nothing more is lost, and (b) less is lost, or at least someone is saved."
>
> Thus, in the case of embryos left over from IVF, research upon which might be useful to saving lives, Outka writes, "They will die, unimplanted in any case. (Nothing more will be lost by their becoming subjects of research.) Thus Outka's conclusion, that, since some lives might be saved, and nothing will be lost, it is permissible to experiment on embryos already alive, but without any hope of being brought to maturation. (10)

In reply, those who are unqualifiedly opposed to embryonic stem cell research point out that "our society does not permit lethal experiments on terminally ill patients or condemned prisoners on the pretext that they will soon die anyway." (7) Similarly, "the fact that an embryonic human being is at risk of being abandoned by his or her parents gives no individual or government a right to directly kill that human being first." (7)

Ethical Issues in Cloning for Stem Cell Research

No sperm is involved in the process of somatic cell nuclear transfer (SCNT). This has raised the question of whether a new human embryo, properly speaking, is produced through this process.

Other opponents of SCNT express concern that it creates human life only to destroy it for research purposes. In fact, no new life is created by SCNT. It works entirely with the ordinary body cells of an already-living person. It no more creates human life than does growing someone's skin cells in tissue culture. . .

SCNT does not entail fertilization of an egg with a sperm. It does not involve conception of a new human life. Instead, it awakens the developmental potential in the genome of cells from a person conceived years ago. (11)

If no new human life is created through SCNT, then the ethical objection that SCNT "creates human life only to destroy it for research purposes" does not hold up.

However, issue is taken with this claim on biological grounds. Critics contend that cloning through SCNT "produces the same result" as fertilization "by combining what is normally combined and activated in fertilization, that is, the full genetic code plus the ovular cytoplasm." (10) That a human embryo is indeed created through SCNT has been affirmed by a prominent embryonic stem cell researcher, James Thomson:

> If you create an embryo by nuclear transfer, and you give it to somebody who didn't know where it came from, there would be no test you could do on that embryo to say where it came from. It is what it is. . . . But by any reasonable definition, at least at some frequency, you're creating an embryo. If you try to define it away, you're being disingenuous. (12)

Further, it is pointed out that SCNT was used to create Dolly the cloned sheep (2), and Dolly was clearly a "new organism." The same procedure of SCNT is used to create an embryo whether it will be used for reproductive purposes or to obtain stem cells. The only difference in the two cases is what is done with the embryo once it is created.

Some who support embryonic stem cell research using embryos left over from IVF treatments have reservations about cloning for stem cell research because of its exploitative impact on women. (13) Thousands, possibly millions of ova will be required for SCNT research (13), and these must be donated by women. Multiple ova, not just one, will be extracted from a woman at a given time. The "extraction of multiple eggs involves both ovarian suppression and what is known as 'ovarian hyperstimulation' using powerful hormones into a woman's body to manipulate it into producing many—often a dozen or more—eggs at a time rather than the normal one or two." (13) However, this procedure can result in ovarian hyperstimulation syndrome (OHSS). In its mild form, OHSS causes symptoms of abdominal discomfort, ovarian enlargement, nausea, and vomiting. In its more severe forms, OHSS can result in loss of fertility, kidney or multiple organ failure, and even death. (13) Ethically, procedures that pose serious risks of harm to persons violate the principle of nonmaleficence. (See chapter 1.) Further, there is concern that SCNT may cause the emergence of a "market in eggs" (13), and that poorer women in need of money may be attracted to egg donation for stem cell research. (14)

Finally, those unqualifiedly opposed to any form of embryonic stem cell research and therapeutic cloning point to demonstrated therapeutic successes using non-embryonic stem cells. (15) It is possible, they contend, to achieve the therapeutic good of stem cell research without the destruction of embryonic life. (16)

CHAPTER SUMMARY

Key Terms and Concepts

stem cell: cells that are capable of dividing and renewing themselves for long periods, are unspecialized, and can give rise to specialized cell types.
somatic cell nuclear transfer (SCNT): a procedure in which the nuclear DNA is removed from an unfertilized ovum and replaced with that of a somatic cell (a non-reproductive body cell) from a donor.
therapeutic cloning: the use of somatic cell nuclear transfer to produce embryonic stem cells that will be a closer match genetically for the intended recipient of the stem cell therapy.

Key Points

- First and foremost, there is intense interest in stem cell research because of therapies that could be developed for a variety of diseases. Embryonic stem cell research could also yield information about human development and insight into serious medical conditions due to abnormal cell division and differentiation. Stem cells could likewise be used to produce differentiated cells for testing new drugs.
- There are various sources of stem cells: embryos, fetuses, adult tissues, umbilical cord blood, amniotic fluid (with the stems cell lodging in the placenta), and menstrual blood. It is likewise possible to genetically reprogram

adult cells to an embryonic stem cell-like state (induced pluripotent stem cells).
- Tissues and organs created from embryonic stem cells will face the problem of immune rejection because they will be genetically different from the recipient. One method that researchers are exploring for overcoming this problem is cloning, using the technique of somatic cell nuclear transfer (SCNT). However, SCNT does not produce an exact genetic match, so that some degree of immune rejection will remain.
- One's judgment about the ethical permissibility of embryonic stem cell research depends on one's views about the status of the early stage embryo, specifically, whether it is a human being with a right to life.
- Even if one considers the early stage embryo to be a human being, some argue that it is still permissible to use spare frozen embryos from fertility clinics in stem cell research because they will be destroyed anyway. Those who are unqualifiedly opposed to embryonic stem cell research point out that our society does not permit lethal experiments on terminally ill patients or condemned prisoners on the grounds that they will soon die anyway.
- Some claim that using somatic cell nuclear transfer (SCNT) to produce stem cells does not involve the creation of a new human embryo properly speaking. However, this claim has been challenged on biological grounds.
- Some who support embryonic stem cell research using embryos left over from IVF treatments have reservations about cloning for stem cell research because of its exploitative impact on women who have to donate the ova to be used in the procedure.

FOR FURTHER DISCUSSION

1. In spite of some opposition, embryonic stem cell research is going forward. From the chapter opening case study, suppose Martha learns that the proposed therapy for her father was developed using embryonic stem cells and that she personally considers embryonic stem cell research to be ethically impermissible. Given that Martha had no part in how the therapy was developed and given its potential for significant benefit for her father, do you think it is ethically permissible for Martha to agree to the use of this therapy even though she regards the way it was developed as ethically wrong?

2. "Some opponents of SCNT contend that it is not pro-life. Former U.S. Senator Jack Danforth, an ordained Episcopal priest with unassailable pro-life credentials, provided the best answer to this concern when he said,

'The proposal to criminalize cell regeneration research calls for a choice between two understandings of human life. On one hand, we have the millions of people who suffer from ALS, Alzheimer's, juvenile diabetes, Parkinson's, spinal cord injuries and cancer—and the loved ones who care for them and suffer by their sides. On the other hand, we have tiny bundles of unfertilized cells existing in Petri dishes. Supporters of the legislation should explain to the afflicted and their loved ones why they care more about those cell bundles than they do about the people.' (11) Do you find this a plausible line of argument? What might opponents of embryonic stem cell research and therapeutic cloning say in response?
3. Research the therapies using non-embryonic stem cells that are currently available. Does this information change your views on embryonic stem cell research?

References

1. National Institutes of Health, *Stem Cell Information: Stem Cell Basics.* http://stemcells.nih.gov/. Accessed April 2009.
2. John Paul II Stem Cell Research Institute, *Stem Cell Education.* http://www.jp2sri.org/. Accessed April 2009.
3. Nikhil Swaminathan, "New Sources of Stem Cells: Amniotic Fluid," *Scientific American* (January 7, 2007). http://www.sciam.com/article.cfm?id=new-source-of-stem-cells. Accessed April 2009.
4. Alison Motluk, "Menstrual blood could be rich source of stem cells." http://www.newscientist.com/article/dn12924-menstrual-blood-cold-be-rich-source-of-stem-cells.html. Accessed April 2009.
5. News@UW-Madison, "Wisconsin scientists culture elusive embryonic stem cells," November 5, 1998. http://www.news.wisconsin.edu/packages/stem-cells. Accessed 2001.
6. NeuroTalk, *Biology 101: An explanation of stem cells and cloning.* http:/neurotalk.psychcentral.com/showthread.php?t=3759. Accessed April 2009.
7. United States Conference of Catholic Bishops, *On Embryonic Stem Cell Research* (2008). http://www.usccb.org. Accessed April 2009.
8. United States Conference of Catholic Bishops, *Ethical and Religious Directives for Catholic Health Care Services* (2001), no. 66. http://www.usccb.org/. Accessed April 2009.
9. "Reproductive Control" in Ronald Munson (ed.), *Intervention and Reflection Basic Issues in Medical Ethics*, 8th ed. (Belmont, CA: Thomson Wadsworth, 2008).

10. Robert P. George and Christopher Tollefsen, *Embryo A Defense of Human Life* (New York: Doubleday, 2008).
11. William B. Neaves, "Stem Cells from Somatic Cell Nuclear Transfer: Research to Unlock the Body's Potential for Self-Repair," *Missouri Medicine* 102/1 (January/February 2005): 14-17, available at http://www.stowers-institute.org/mediacenter/docs/NeavesSomaticCellFeature.pdf. Accessed April 2009.
12. Alan Boyle, "Stem cell pioneer does a reality check: James Thomson on science and morality," http://www.msnbc.msn.com/id/8303756. Accessed April 2009.
13. Diane Beeson, Testimony to the House Government Reform Subcommittee on Criminal Justice, Drug Policy and Human Resources – Hearing on Stem Cell Research (March 7, 2006). http://www.handsoffourovaries.com/. Accessed April 2009.
14. Core European Seminar: Human Egg Trading and the Exploitation of Women (Brussels, June 30, 2005). http://www.handsoffourovaries.com/. Accessed April 2009.
15. Do No Harm The Coalition of Americans for Research Ethics. http://www.stemcellresearch.org/. Accessed April 2009.
16. *The Science of Stem Cells Finding Cures and Protecting Life*. Michigan Catholic Conference, DVD.

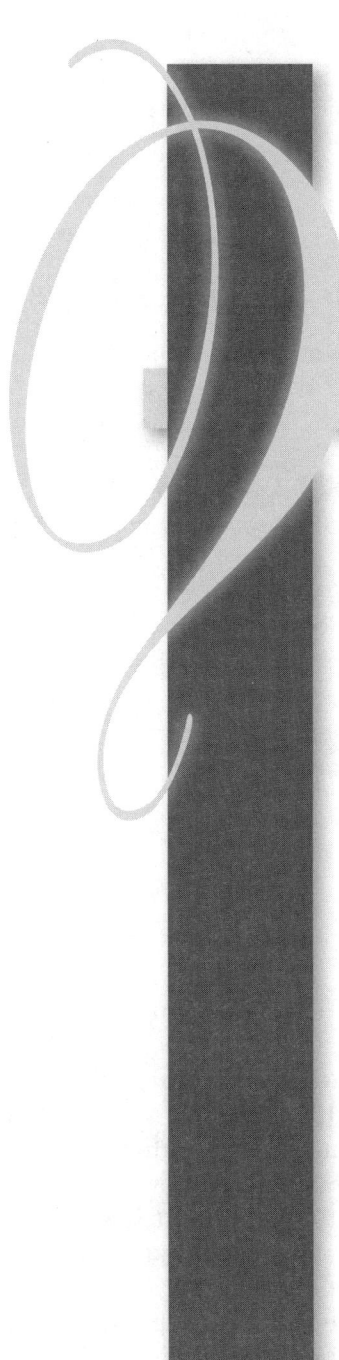

Chapter 17

Issues in Organ Procurement and Allocation

When obtaining or renewing a driver's license, you may be asked if you wish to be an organ donor if death should occur. This is one of the measures being used to try to increase the number of organ donors since many more patients are in need of organ transplants at any given time than the number of organs actually available for transplant. (1) This fact of a discrepancy between patient need and available resources raises yet another issue. Once an organ becomes available for transplant, how do we fairly decide who should receive it? This is a particularly weighty question because, in making the allocation decision, we may literally be deciding who lives and who dies. (2)

In this chapter you will learn about:

- standards for determining death and the relation of these standards to organ procurement;

- actual and proposed ways of recruiting organ donors;
- criteria and principles for deciding on the distribution of organs to particular patients.

Case Study

Berta Romero has worked as a respiratory therapist at Lakeland Community Hospital for ten years. She has been involved in removing ventilators from dying patients on many occasions. However, an incident occurred recently which left her feeling "shaken."

Berta was paged to come to a room near the hospital's surgery center. In it she found a patient on a ventilator. She was told that the patient was dying and had been moved to this room from the ICU. The ventilator would be removed and, as soon as the patient's heart stopped, she would be taken into surgery to remove organs for transplantation purposes.

Berta has always been an advocate of organ donation. However, this procedure makes her feel like a "vulture." Is it right, she wonders, to deliberately choose to let a patient die at a particular time in order that her organs can be taken for transplantation to others?

Determining Death and Organ Procurement

Living persons can donate some organs and tissues—such as kidneys, a segment of the liver, a lobe of the lung, and portions of the intestine and pancreas. (3) From an ethical point of view, a living donor can "give organs whose removal will not adversely affect his or her ability to live in a relatively healthy state." (4)

All organs and tissues that can be transplanted can be obtained from those who are deceased. (4) In the latter case, the *dead donor rule* is currently followed; that is, organs cannot be taken for transplant purposes until the patient has reliably been pronounced dead. (4) Thus the practice of organ transplantation leads us into the question of the definition and determination of death.

Today, two different standards for determining death are widely accepted. An individual may be declared dead who has sustained *either* the irreversible cessation of circulatory and respiratory functions *or* the irreversible cessation of all functions of the entire brain, including the brainstem ("whole brain death").

(4) The first is a cardiopulmonary criterion of death, and the second, a neurological criterion. (4)

In the case scenario involving respiratory therapist Berta Romero, the patient's organs would be retrieved for transplant purposes after the patient's heart stopped beating. However, special problems are posed in using such non-heart-beating donors:

> A key challenge to procuring organs from non-heart-beating cadavers is posed by warm ischemic damage, caused by the lack of blood perfusion while the organs are still in the body of the newly deceased donor. To prevent or limit this damage, the time between the cessation of circulation ("effective asystole") and the procurement of organs must be minimized. For this purpose, the final cardiac contractions must be *controlled:* In the moments following asystole, the body must be prepared for surgeons either to remove the organs promptly or to maintain their viability for transplantation in the ensuing hours. For the moment of cardiac arrest to be controlled in this way, the prospective organ donor must be a patient from whom a ventilator and perhaps other forms of life-sustaining treatment will be withdrawn, either in accordance with the patient's wishes or the wishes of a surrogate. In other words, a potential non-heart-beating donor, in the vast majority of cases, is an individual who is ventilator-dependent but not yet deceased according to today's neurological standard. The ventilator is then removed, the patient is watched and kept comfortable until the heart stops circulating blood through the body, a waiting period is observed (usually two to five minutes), and then the surgical procurement of organs begins. (4)

The practice of *controlled donation after cardiac death* raises various questions. Following the dead donor rule, can we be sure that the patient is in fact dead when the procedure of organ retrieval is begun? How long should we wait after the patient's heart has stopped before the retrieval procedure is started? Could the patient have been resuscitated and brought back to life? In order to secure an organ for transplant, will life-sustaining treatment (such as a ventilator) be withdrawn too soon? Overall, will good quality end-of-life care be compromised for the patient-donor? (4)

Thus it has been proposed that "a morally sound hospital policy" on planned donation after cardiac death should include the following stipulations (5):

- The decision to withdraw medical interventions must be made independently of the decision to donate an organ.

- Organ donors must receive the same end-of-life palliative care as non-donors.
- The hospital should provide the donor's family with the option of being present when life support is withdrawn and, in general, take every measure to permit family and friends to say goodbye in a dignified way.
- Procurement teams must wait the recommended amount of time after the permanent cessation of heart function before beginning the removal of organs.
- The medical staff overseeing withdrawal of medical interventions must not hasten the patient's death, even if the organs might become unusable for transplantation.
- If patients do not die quickly enough to become donors, they should be returned to the intensive care unit to die in a peaceful and respectful way. (5)

Incorporating such stipulations into hospital policy on organ retrieval should work against a view of planned donation after cardiac death as nothing more than "letting patients die so that their organs can be used for transplant."

Recruiting Organ Donors

The United States currently operates under a system of *altruistic donation* of organs and tissues. Individuals (or their family or proxy decision maker) must voluntarily make the choice to donate organs and tissues, without compensation. However, under the current system of altruistic donation there is a serious shortage of needed organs. (6) Some contend that the "current altruistic system has not failed as much as it has not been fully promoted" in that many potential donor families are simply never asked about donating the organs of their deceased relative. (6) At the same time, various alternative programs have been proposed to increase organ donation.

One proposal is to provide *financial incentives* for organ donation. For example, an individual might agree in advance to donate organs upon death, with payment to beneficiaries or to his estate occurring after donation has taken place. (6) Or again, organ donation might be accompanied by a set reimbursement for funeral expenses (6), or tax credits might be provided to the donor or to his family. (7) If a system of financial incentives increases the supply of organs, such incentives would be justified by the saving of lives which would otherwise be lost. (6) Further, it is argued that "some form of compensation is the right thing to do" because, at present, "the donor and the family are the only participants not directly benefitting from the process" of organ donation. (6)

From an ethical point of view, there is concern that providing financial incentives for organ donation may lead to decreased respect for life and the sanctity of the human body (6), with the human body becoming "a commodity to be bought, sold and bartered for in a manner similar to any other good or service." (6) There is also a danger that financial incentives for organ donation could coerce the poor into agreeing to donate their organs. (6) Moreover, there is fear that a system of financial reimbursement for organ donation would create an atmosphere in society downgrading the virtue of altruism. (8)

An alternative proposal is granting *preferred status* for organ donors. In other words, "individuals who have signified their intention to be organ/tissue donors...would receive points or other value that would somewhat facilitate the likelihood of receiving an organ, should they need it in the future." (9) This benefit might also extend to "first degree relatives of those who have signed up or have actually been donors." (9) An argument in favor of granting preferred status is based on justice. Specifically, "is it fair for an individual who is willing to participate in the system of transplantation to not receive an organ while another medically similar individual who was unwilling to participate receives a transplant?" (9) Further, unlike providing financial incentives for organ donation, preferred status is equitable across economic strata of society; the value of a life-giving organ is the same to a very poor disadvantaged person as to someone who is wealthy. (9) At the same time, there are practical difficulties in determining fairly the weight to be given to the intention to be an organ donor. (9) For example, it might be a tie-breaker, other things being equal (9), but it "should probably not be sufficient to place an elective case with a short time on the list ahead of one who is about to die, or who has been waiting for years." (9)

Another possible approach to organ donation is *presumed consent*. Under this system, a "candidate for cadaveric organ and tissue recovery is presumed to have consented to organ and tissue recovery if he or she has not registered a refusal." (10) This approach is grounded on our duty to promote the good of society. (10)

> The communitarian view holds that individuals have a moral duty to help others when the cost to the individual of helping is very low. Since cadaveric organ donation can save the lives of others and causes no significant harm to the decedent or the family, individuals who do not object on religious grounds have a moral duty to donate their organs. (11)

At the same time, this approach respects individual autonomy "by giving objectors to organ donation an opportunity to empower their anti-donation preference." (10) Further, presumed consent would eliminate the need to ask the donor's family for consent at a time when the family is grieving. (10) Concerns about presumed consent focus on the practical difficulties of ensuring that all who object to organ donation in fact have the opportunity to register their refusal with public authorities, and setting up the mechanisms for registering and transmitting objection status. (10)

Yet another proposal for increasing organ donation is known as *required response* or *mandated choice*. (10, 11) Under this system, all adults would be required by public authorities to express their preferences regarding organ donation (that is, their willingness to donate or objection to donation) when, for example, they renew their driver's licenses, file income tax forms, or perform some other task mandated by the state. (10, 11) These preferences would be recorded in a national donor registry. (10) This approach is supported by research indicating that the primary reason more people do not sign organ donor cards is because of the fact that no authority has asked them. (10) From an ethical point of view, this approach respects the value of individual autonomy as all adult persons make a decision for or against organ donation. (10)

Once organs or tissues are available for transplant, the question must be faced of who should receive them since there are many more people in need of transplants than there are organs and tissues available. This is the issue to which we now turn.

Case Study

Allen Potter is a lab technician at Mercy Medical Center. He has been asked to do three lab tests—bilirubin, INR, and creatinine—for Sam Langan in preparation for placing him on the waiting list for a liver transplant. (12)

Sam is 68, and a prominent attorney in the community. He is still active in his church, and has served several terms on the school board. He is currently chair of the annual United Way fund drive. However, throughout his life Sam has struggled with the problem of heavy drinking, which is the reason he needs a liver transplant. Two years ago he voluntarily entered a rehab program, and has had his drinking under control since that time.

Allen Potter has no doubt in his mind that Sam is "worthy" of a liver transplant. He has been, and continues to be, a valuable member of the community. Allen has heard stories of some people waiting for years to get an organ, while others seem to get them almost immediately. Allen hopes Sam can get a transplant before he becomes too debilitated, or even dies.

■ ■ ■

Allocating Organs to Transplant Recipients

Developing a method for allocating organs among possible recipients is a work in progress. Changes and refinements in procedures are ongoing. We will describe various allocation procedures that have been used.

In the case of living organ donors, donation may be *directed* or *non-directed.* In directed donation, the organ donor specifies the recipient of the organ. For example, blood relatives of the transplant candidate, such as parents, brothers or sisters, or adult children, may engage in directed donation. Directed donation may also be used by persons who have some type of social connection with the transplant candidate, such as a spouse or significant other, a friend, or a co-worker. Acquaintances of the transplant candidate, or even strangers who have learned about the transplant candidate, may also engage in directed donation. On the other hand, non-directed donation occurs when individuals donate to an unspecified, anonymous candidate on the transplant waiting list. (3)

A particular type of directed donation is *paired donation* or *paired exchange.* This arrangement involves two pairs e.g., of living kidney donors and transplant candidates who have incompatible blood types, with the two transplant candidates "trading" donors. (3) This arrangement is easiest to understand through an example:

> Barbara wants to donate to her sister Donna, but they do not have compatible blood types. Carlos wants to donate to his wife Maria, but they are also not compatible. By "swapping" donors so that Carlos matches Donna and Barbara matches Maria, two transplants are made possible. (3)

This type of arrangement can also involve multiple living donor and transplant candidate pairs. (3)

Yet another arrangement available to living donors is *donor waiting list exchange.* For example, a living donor who has an incompatible blood type with the intended kidney transplant candidate will donate to an anonymous candidate on the waiting list, with the intended transplant candidate in turn being given higher priority on the waiting list. (3)

In the case of directed donation to a relative by blood or marriage or to a significant other, the practice of directed donation can be justified ethically by appealing to the intuition that we have stronger obligations to persons with whom we are in special relationships than to strangers. (13) The practice of directed donation can also be justified on utilitarian grounds (see chapter 1); namely, that it makes more organs available for transplant and hence saves additional lives (assuming that the donor would not be inclined to donate to an anonymous recipient). What has been ethically controversial, however, is the direction of organs to a specific social group; for example, to a group defined by race, religion, ethnicity, gender, or sexual orientation. (13) In one recorded case, a man who was a sympathizer of the Ku Klux Klan was shot and killed in a robbery. His family agreed to donate his organs, but stipulated "donation to White recipients only." (13) Directed donation to a particular social group has been opposed on the grounds that it represents "unequal treatment based on morally irrelevant considerations." (13)

The case study involving Sam Langan concerns transplant of a liver most probably to be obtained from a cadaver. At one point, the United Network for Organ Sharing (UNOS) adopted the principle that donated livers should go to the patient most urgently in need at the time that a transplantable liver becomes available. (12) The following procedure was used for making allocation decisions for individuals aged 12 or older:

- Status 1 patients are those who have acute (sudden and severe onset) liver failure and a life expectancy of hours to a few days without a transplant.
- Other candidates for liver transplants are given a score between 6 (less ill) and 40 (gravely ill) based on how urgently the candidate needs a transplant within the next three months, as calculated by a formula using three lab test results.
- If the donor is younger than 18, then the following prioritization scheme is used:
  — The liver is given first to a Status 1 patient.
  — The liver is offered next to candidates age 11 or younger in the geographical region.
  — The liver is then made available to candidates with a score of 15 or higher, locally and then regionally, with patients aged 12 to 17 considered ahead of adult patients.
- If the donor is 18 or older, then the following prioritization scheme is used:
  — The liver is given first to Status 1 candidates, locally and regionally.
  — The liver is offered next to candidates with a score of 15 or higher, locally and then regionally.
  — The liver is then made available to candidates with a score of 14 or less, locally and then regionally.
  — Finally, the liver is made available to any compatible candidates nationwide, beginning with Status 1 candidates and then to those with the highest scores.
- The time of a transplant candidate on the waiting list is considered only when there are two or more transplant candidates with the same blood type and score. (12)

In sum, the criteria used for allocating livers for transplant purposes include urgency of need, age, geographical location, and time on the transplant waiting list.

UNOS has used somewhat different criteria for allocating different organs. In the case of lung transplants, the patient's "score" has been "an estimate of the severity of each candidate's illness and his or her chance of success following a lung transplant." (14) Their kidney allocation policy has taken into account the length of time spent on the waiting list, whether the potential organ candidate is a child, the body size of both the donor and the transplant candidate, blood type, and blood antibody levels. (15)

From an ethical point of view, the allocation of organs has been described in terms of balancing two values: *efficiency* in the use of organs and *fairness* in distribution (i.e., justice or equity). (16) From a justice perspective, concern has been raised about the use of geographical criteria for allocating organs.

The aforementioned scheme for allocating liver transplants contains stipulations prioritizing allocation at local, regional, and national levels. In defense of granting priority at the local level, it may be argued that such prioritization will make people more willing to donate organs because "it is natural for each community to feel it should serve its own members first" and because people "like to think that they are helping their neighbors." (13) It may also be argued that granting priority at the local level helps maintain the quality of organs by keeping ischemia times brief and further, that it supports local transplant centers which enable patients to be transplanted close to home. (13) On the other hand, geographical prioritization at local and regional levels may entail the inequity of "directing organs to healthier patients over those who are desperately ill simply because of the morally irrelevant variable of where one happens to live." (13) Or again, such geographical prioritization may result in unequal waiting times for an organ for patients with equal severity of illness. (13) Such inequities are brought forward as reasons for establishing a single *national* list for organ transplantation. (13) The only recognized exception in which organs could be "restricted solely on the basis of geographical proximity between the donor and the recipient" would be "those cases in which medical necessity prohibits transport of the organ in a way that would maintain viability." (13)

In our case study the transplant candidate, Sam Langan, is 68 years old. Should his age be a factor in prioritizing him for a liver transplant? Intuitively, we may well feel that an 80-year-old should not have the same priority for an organ transplant as someone who is 20, or 30, or 40 years old. But what about someone who is 68?

Ethicists have proposed different positions on the appropriateness of considering age as one factor figuring into allocation of organs for transplant. One view is that "the elderly deserve equal treatment" with other candidates. (13)

The reason is that "justice requires treating similarly situated people equally and that those who are sickest deserve priority even if it is not always the most efficient use of resources." (13) Thus "all persons who are equally sick, regardless of age, deserve equal treatment." (13) A contrasting view works with the concept of *justice-over-a-lifetime:*

> It asks who is worst off considering people's whole lives. From the moment-in-time perspective, a 40-year-old and a 70-year-old dying of heart failure are equally poor off, but considering their entire lives who could deny that the one who was healthy enough to make it to 70 is much better off? To be fair, we need to allocate our resources so that the 40-year-old has a chance to make it to 70. From this over-a-lifetime perspective, justice requires that we target organs for these younger persons who are so poorly off that they will not make it to old age without being given special priority. The younger the age of the person needing an organ, the higher the claim. (13)

In other words, on this scheme entitlement to organs would be inversely proportional to age, and this factor would apply regardless of where one is in the life span. (13) Further, this standard "would provide a smooth, gradual priority inversely related to age rather than producing a precipitous drop off in entitlement at some birthday." (13) Thus, applied to the case of someone like Sam Langan at age 68, the justice-over-a-lifetime standard would take his age into account as a factor lessening his entitlement to a transplant without totally precluding the possibility of an organ transplant for him.

In the case study Sam Langan's need for a liver transplant has been caused by heavy drinking. Behaviors such as drinking alcohol, smoking cigarettes, eating fatty foods, and a failure to exercise increase the likelihood of needing an organ transplant. (13) Ethically, the question has been raised of whether persons engaging in such behaviors have less claim to an organ transplant in a prioritization scheme, or even whether they should be totally excluded from eligibility. Before giving an affirmative answer to this question, it is critical to determine the extent to which such behaviors are voluntary and the extent to which genetic, psychological, and economic factors play a causal role. (13) However, this is not an easy task and the answer is not clear cut. The Ethics and Social Impact Committee of the Transplant and Health Policy Center in Ann Arbor, Michigan, has argued that, even if alcoholism involves an ethically blameworthy weakness of will, it is not legitimate to categorically deny liver transplants to alcoholics suffering from end-stage cirrhosis. (17) They point out that, as a general rule, we do not engage in moral evaluation of transplant candidates as a condition for eligibility: "We do not seek to determine whether a particular transplant candidate is an abusive parent or a dutiful daughter, whether candidates cheat on their income taxes or their spouses, or whether potential recipients pay their parking tickets or routinely lie when they think it is in their best interests." (17) Similarly, an alcoholic should not be subjected to personal moral scrutiny as a condition for receiving an organ transplant.

In the case scenario the lab technician Allen Potter considers Sam Langan a "worthy" candidate for an organ transplant because of his social contributions. Sam is a prominent attorney, is active in his church, has served several terms on the school board and is currently chair of the annual United Way fund drive. The rationale for taking into account the social worth of a potential organ recipient might be this: if society invests a scarce resource in one person rather than another, society has a right to consider what it will receive in return. (18) However, judging someone's social worth in making organ allocation decisions has proven very controversial because of the subjective nature of the judgments involved. Many would not want this to be a factor in allocating organs for transplantation. (19)

CHAPTER SUMMARY

Key Terms and Concepts

brain death: the death of a person as determined by the irreversible cessation of all brain functions.
cardiopulmonary death: the death of a person as determined by the irreversible cessation of circulatory and respiratory functions.
controlled donation after cardiac death: a practice of coordinating the withdrawal of life-sustaining treatment with organ retrieval so as to allow prompt retrieval of organs after cardiopulmonary death has occurred.
presumed consent: a candidate for cadaveric organ and tissue recovery is presumed to have consented to organ and tissue recovery if he or she has not registered a refusal.
required response/mandated choice: all adults would be required by public authorities to express their preferences regarding organ donation, either their willingness to donate or objection to donation.
directed organ donation: the organ donor specifies the recipient of the organ.
non-directed organ donation: the donor donates to an unspecified, anonymous candidate on the transplant waiting list.

Key Points

- Living persons can donate some organs and tissues. All organs and tissues that can be transplanted can be obtained from those who are deceased.
- The dead donor rule affirms that, in the case of cadaveric organ and tissue recovery, organs cannot be taken for transplant purposes until the patient has actually been pronounced dead.
- Two different standards are commonly used for determining death: cardiopulmonary death and brain death.
- There are special challenges, medically and ethically, in the case of non-heart-beating organ donation. This practice requires safeguards to be put into place.
- The United States currently operates under a system of *voluntary donation* of organs and tissues. However, this system has left us with an acute shortage of organs for transplantation. Proposed methods for increasing organ donation include offering financial incentives, granting preferred status to receive an organ to those agreeing to donate (or to their families), presuming consent to donate organs, and requiring people to make an explicit choice for or against organ donation. Ethical principles and values are important in evaluating these proposals.
- From an ethical point of view, the allocation of organs has been described in terms of balancing two values: *efficiency* in the use of organs and *fairness* in distribution (i.e., justice or equity).
- There are ethical questions regarding the use of geographical location, age, behavioral responsibility for one's disease, or social worth as criteria in allocating organs for transplantation.

FOR FURTHER DISCUSSION

1. Have you ever been present when someone died? What made you believe or feel that the person was dead? How do your intuitions about what constitutes death compare with the brain death criterion? With the cardiopulmonary criterion?
2. Have you signed an organ donor card? Why or why not? Share and discuss your responses.
3. Suppose that your sister (or brother), with whom you are quite close, needs a kidney transplant. You are told that you are a good match. You are told

that the risks of serious complications following removal of one kidney are rare; the donor's kidney function rapidly returns to approximately 90 percent of what it was before surgery. Nevertheless, should the donor's remaining kidney become diseased or injured later in life, there will be serious consequences for the donor. (20)

- *Under these conditions, would you agree to donate one of your kidneys to your sister (or brother)? Why or why not?*
- *Would you feel pressured to donate a kidney by family ties? How do you think your sister (or brother) would react if you declined to donate? How do you think your parents would react if you declined to donate?*

4. Aborted fetuses have been considered a possible source of organs for transplant purposes. Suppose that someone who desperately needs a kidney transplant finds that he could benefit by receiving a kidney from an aborted fetus (21). Let us suppose further that the patient in question personally is ethically opposed to abortion. In good conscience, can he accept the kidney from an aborted fetus as an organ transplant for himself?
5. Parents have a child in need of a bone marrow transplant. Suppose that they decide to conceive another child to try to provide a compatible donor. There is no intention of abortion; rather, this second child will be brought to birth and be raised in the family. (22) Is their course of action permissible from an ethical point of view?
6. In the future it may be possible to clone a particular person in order to provide a compatible source of organs and tissues for transplant purposes. (23) Do you think this would be an ethically acceptable use of human cloning?
7. A *xenograft* is the transfer of tissue or organs between individuals of different species. A famous case of cross-species transplantation occurred at Loma Linda University Medical Center when the defective heart of "Baby Fae" was replaced with the heart of a baboon. The infant lived twenty days before rejecting the heart. (24) Experimentation with transplantation of animal organs into humans is likely to continue in the future. Do you see any ethical issues with transplanting animal organs into humans?
8. In general, we do not consider social worth as an appropriate criterion to use in making decisions about allocating organs for transplant. However, suppose that a prison inmate, who has been convicted of a serious crime, is in need of an organ transplant. Should the prisoner be considered ineligible for an organ transplant because of his harmful actions against society?

References

1. United Network for Organ Sharing, "Waiting list candidates." http://www.unos.org. Accessed May 2009.
2. National Kidney Foundation, "25 Facts about Organ Donation and Transplantation." http://www.kidney.org/news/newsroom/fs_new/25factsorgdon&trans.cfm. Accessed May 2009.
3. United Network for Organ Sharing, *Living Donation Information you need to know.* http://www.unos.org/SharedContentDocuments/Living_Donation_Booklet_Final.pdf. Accessed May 2009.
4. The President's Council on Bioethics, *Controversies on the Determination of Death* (January 2009). http://bioethicsprint.bioethics.gov/reports/death/. Accessed May 2009.
5. Sam Crowe and Eric Cohen, *Organ Transplantation: Potential Policy Recommendations:* A Staff Working Paper of the President's Council on Bioethics. http://www.bioethics.gov/background/organ_recs.html. Accessed May 2009.
6. Edward W. Nelson, James E. Childress, Jennie Perryman, Victor Robards, Albert Rowan, Michael W. Seely, Sylvester Sterioff, and Mary Rovelli Swanson, *Financial Incentives for Organ Donation:* A Report of the Payment Subcommittee, United Network for Organ Sharing Ethics Committee (1993). http://www.unos.org/resources/bioethics.asp. Accessed May 2009.
7. Arthur L. Caplan, "Organ Procurement: It's Not in the Cards," *Hastings Center Report* 14/5 (October 1984): 9-12.
8. Kathryn Schroeter, "The Ethics of Organ Donation," *Today's O.R. Nurse* (January/February 1995): 8-12.
9. James F. Burdick, Alexander M. Capron, Francis L. Delmonico, Mark D. Ravenscraft, Craig R. Reckhard, and Michael Shapiro, *Preferred Status for Organ Donors:* A Report of the United Network for Organ Sharing Ethics Committee (1993). http://www.unos.org/resources/bioethics.asp. Accessed May 2009.
10. J. Michael Dennis, Patricia Hanson, Ernest Hodge, Ruud A.F. Krom, and Robert M. Veatch, *An Evaluation of the Ethics of Presumed Consent and A Proposal Based on Required Response* A Report of the Presumed Consent Subcommittee, United Network for Organ Sharing Ethics Committee (1993). http://www.unos.org/resources/bioethics.asp. Accessed May 2009.
11. Council on Ethical and Judicial Affairs of the American Medical Association, "Strategies for Cadaveric Organ Procurement," *Journal of the American Medical Association* 272/10 (September 14, 1994): 809-12.

12. United Network for Organ Sharing, *Questions and Answers for Transplant Candidates about MELD and PELD.* http://www.unos.org/SharedContentDocuments/MELD_PELD(1).pdf. Accessed May 2009.
13. Robert M. Veatch, *Transplantation Ethics* (Washington, DC: Georgetown University Press, 2000).
14. United Network for Organ Sharing, *Questions and Answers for Transplant Candidates about Lung Allocation Policy.* http://www.unos.org/SharedContentDocuments/Lung_Patient(1).pdf. Accessed May 2009.
15. United Network for Organ Sharing, *Information for Kidney Transplant Candidates and their Families.* http://www.unos.org/SharedContentDocuments/ExpandedCriteriaDonor_KidneysBrochure.pdf. Accessed May 2009.
16. F. Daniel Davis, "The Ethics of Organ Allocation: Policy Questions Concerning Geography, Age, and Net Benefit," A Staff Discussion Paper of the President's Council on Bioethics (2007). http://www.bioethics.gov/background/ethics_of_organ_allocation.html. Accessed May 2009.
17. Carl Cohen, Martin Benjamin, and the Ethics and Social Impact Committee of the Transplant and Health Policy Center, Ann Arbor, Michigan, "Alcoholics and Liver Transplantation," *Journal of the American Medical Association* 265 (March 13, 1991): 1299-1301.
18. Nichols Rescher, "The Allocation of Exotic Medical Lifesaving Technology," *Ethics* 79/3 (April 1969): 173-86.
19. *Doctor, I Want . . .* , Hard Choices Series, KCTS/Seattle, 1980, video.
20. Karen K. Giuliano, "Organ Transplants: Tackling the Tough Ethical Questions," *Nursing* (May 1997): 34-40.
21. "Can the Fetus be an Organ Farm?" in Carol Levine and Robert M. Veatch (eds.), *Cases in Bioethics from the Hastings Center Report* (Hastings-on-Hudson, NY: The Hastings Center, 1982).
22. "Case Presentation: Saviour Sibling" in Ronald Munson (ed.), *Intervention and Reflection Basic Issues in Medical Ethics*, 8th ed. (Belmont, CA: Thomson Wadsworth, 2008).
23. President's Council on Bioethics, *Human Cloning and Human Dignity* (New York: Public Affairs, 2002).
24. Ricki Lewis, *Human Genetics: Concepts and Applications*, 2nd ed. (Dubuque, IA: Wm C. Brown Publishers, 1997).

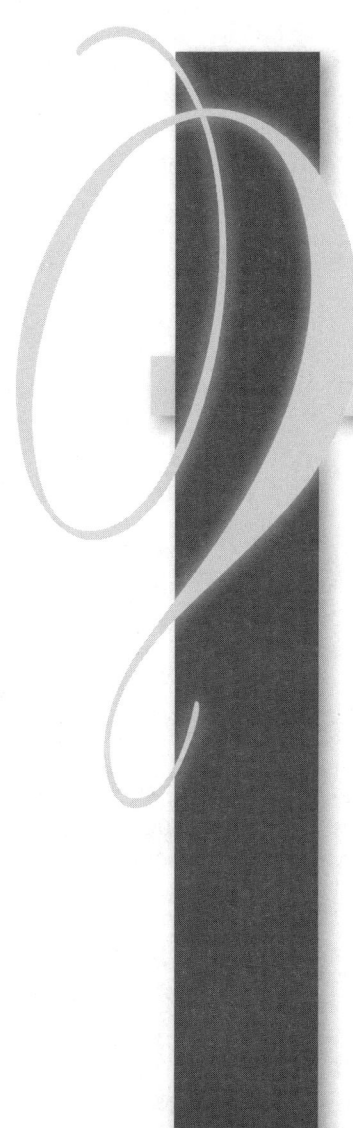

Chapter 18

Genetics in the 21st Century: The DNA Frontier

A landmark scientific enterprise of the late twentieth century was the *Human Genome Project* (HGP). Coordinated by the U.S. Department of Energy and the National Institutes of Health, this thirteen year project had as goals the identification of all the genes in human DNA as well as determination of the sequences of the three billion chemical base pairs that make up human DNA. Although the HGP was completed in 2003, analyses of the data collected will continue for many years. (1) This new knowledge "about the make-up and functioning of the chemical building blocks of human life will give rise to insights into the causes and pathways of numerous diseases that inflict untold suffering upon humanity," in turn "making possible opportunities for more effective diagnosis, prevention, and treatment of many diseases." (2)

Allied health professionals have already become involved in the realm of genetics in providing health care services. They have found themselves in the position of taking family histories of the occurrence of diseases, discussing the genetic basis of disorders and correcting the misconceptions of patients, and making referrals for genetic services. (3) In fact, a field in allied health has emerged called the "genetic associate." (4, 5)

In this chapter you will learn about:

- the ELSI project in genetics;
- the pros and cons of undertaking presymptomatic genetic testing;
- genetic discrimination and health insurance.

Case Study

Tom Morris provides physical therapy for James McDonald, a man in his early forties who has developed the symptoms of Huntington's disease. HD is an adult-onset genetic disorder that causes uncontrollable movements and personality changes. (6)

Tom finds it somewhat disturbing to take care of Mr. McDonald because it reminds him of a genetic disease in his own family. His grandfather developed Alzheimer's disease at age 69 and Tom remembers vividly the progressive deterioration of his grandfather over a period of ten years before he died, and how he had to be placed in a special unit at a nursing home because he was so "out of it." Recently Tom's own father, who is only 66, has been diagnosed with Alzheimer's disease. His father's older brother is also suspected of having Alzheimer's.

The university medical center at which Tom works has a genetic counseling center. From talking with a genetic associate, Tom knows that he could undergo testing to determine if he has inherited the allele (that is, the form of the gene) for Alzheimer's disease. Tom has two older sisters who would be candidates for genetic testing as well because of the family history of Alzheimer's.

Tom is ambivalent about undergoing genetic testing. He worries about receiving a positive test result. He is only 26 and is engaged to be married in a few months. He doesn't want a cloud hanging over his life that he will develop a devastating disease at some point. Quite frankly, the thought of ending up like his grandfather scares him. Moreover, Tom recently read a feature article in a newspaper about "genetic discrimination." It related the case of a woman who was terminated from her job a month after she shared with her employer the information of a positive test result for HD. (7) The old saying "Ignorance is bliss," Tom thinks, seems like good advice to follow in this situation.

■ ■ ■

ELSI

Accompanying the human genome project is ELSI, a project looking at the *ethical, legal, and social implications* of current work in the field of genetics. (8) Four areas have been identified as requiring discussion and reflection among health care professionals and patients: privacy and fair use of genetic information; responsible clinical integration of genetic information; stigmatization and discrimination based on genetic traits; and professional and public education. (9)

The following is a sampling of more specific questions arising in each of these general categories.

Privacy and Fair Use of Genetic Information

- Should genetic information be treated differently from other medical information in reports, charts, or other medical records?
- Should written informed consent be obtained from clients before their genetic information is shared with third parties?
- After taking a genetic test, should clients have the right not to be told the results?

Clinical Integration of Genetic Information

- Should health care professionals provide patients and families with developmental prognoses based on genetic screening results?
- Should patients be able to have their children tested for genetic conditions that do not show symptoms until adulthood if the conditions are neither treatable nor preventable?

- If a health care professional suspects that a patient has a genetic condition that is not diagnosed, does he or she have a professional obligation to share this information? If so, with whom?

Preventing Stigmatization and Discrimination Based on Genetic Traits

- What role should society have to ensure fairness in the use of genetic information by both insurers and employers?
- What role should professionals have in helping to prevent stigmatization of people with genetic conditions?
- What are some of the racial/ethnic issues in genetics that professionals should consider?

Professional and Public Education

- What should professional associations do to help ensure their members' professional competence in the new genetics?
- What role should health care professionals have in educating their patients about the implications of genetics? (9)

In considering the case study involving Tom Morris and his family history of Alzheimer's disease, we will focus on issues surrounding genetic testing and on genetic discrimination in health insurance.

Genetic Testing

The case of Tom Morris involves *presymptomatic* genetic testing; that is, testing to determine if an individual carries a form of a gene that is related to the occurrence of a particular disease before the individual actually starts to show symptoms of the disease. (10) What benefits are there to engaging in presymptomatic genetic testing? Psychologically, individuals report a sense of relief from the uncertainty of not knowing their status. This reaction may hold true even when a positive test result is expected (and received). (10) Further, if a positive test result is received, the individual can make plans for the future. This might include decisions about type of job, selection of preferred health care facilities, and decisions about having children. (10) Very important to consider is the usefulness of the information gained through a genetic test. In some cases an individual who tests positive may be able to take steps to prevent or delay the onset of the symptoms of the disease. (11)

On the other hand, receiving a positive test result can have a negative psychological impact. Some individuals have reported feelings of "emotional numbness, sadness, depression, and anger." (10) An individual who has tested positive may fear loss of employment and health insurance, and may experience a sense of guilt over the possibility of having transmitted the genetic disorder to his or her children. (10) Further, even receiving the good news of a negative test result may not be free of harmful consequences. If an individual has tested negative while other family members have tested positive, he may experience guilt over his good fortune in comparison to the fate of other family members. (10)

Thus decisions about undergoing genetic testing involve a balancing of pros and cons. In our case study, Tom Morris is a young adult who "doesn't want a cloud hanging over his life that he will develop a devastating disease at some point." He has seen the effects of Alzheimer's disease on his grandfather and "the thought of ending up like his grandfather scares him." Indeed, he even finds it "somewhat disturbing" to provide physical therapy services for a man with a genetic disease because it reminds him of his own family history of Alzheimer's. Thus a positive test result for Tom would likely have a very adverse effect on him psychologically. Moreover, Tom is aware of the possibility of experiencing genetic discrimination through a newspaper article he has read. All of these considerations argue against Tom undertaking presymptomatic genetic testing for Alzheimer's disease. But are there any countervailing considerations? Are there any reasons in favor of Tom undertaking genetic testing that might outweigh these arguments against it? To answer this question, we must consider further the genetics of Alzheimer's disease.

Genes known to be involved in the development of Alzheimer's disease include amyloid precursor protein (APP) on chromosome 21, presenilin 1 (PS1) on chromosome14, presenilin 2 (PS2) on chromosome 1, and apolipoprotein E (APOE) on chromosome 19. The first three genes are associated with early-onset autosomal-dominant Alzheimer's disease. (12, 13, 14, 15) "Early-onset" means that the symptoms of Alzheimer's disease start before the age of 55. (16) To say that the gene is "dominant" means that the gene will be expressed—that is, that a person with this gene will almost certainly develop the symptoms of Alzheimer's disease. However, there are limitations in testing for these genes, as this example illustrates:

> Carrying a mutation in PS1 . . . confers near certainty of developing AD. However, mutations in PS1 are found in only a small fraction of all AD

cases. . . . Thus, while the predictive value is high, the usefulness of this test for most people is limited: a vast majority of the people who develop AD would test negative for PS1 mutations. (12)

The variant (allele) of the APOE gene known as "e4" confers a susceptibility to late-onset Alzheimer's disease (15)—that is, to the occurrence of the disease after age 65. (16) It should be carefully noted that having APOE e4 does not guarantee development of Alzheimer's disease; rather, it is a *susceptibility* gene that makes the development of Alzheimer's disease more likely. Whether an individual with this type of gene will in fact develop Alzheimer's disease may be influenced by environmental factors, such as "a history of head trauma with loss of consciousness . . . and low levels of education and socioeconomic status." (15) There are again limitations surrounding the test for this type of gene:

> Apolipoprotein E e4 used as a screening test for AD is neither sensitive nor specific. At least half of patients with AD have no e4 allele; many with this allele never develop the disease. . . . One further complication in using APOE e4 as a screening test may be found in the concept of residual risk, the risk that remains after a negative test result. Even if an individual is found through screening to have no copies of e4, he or she is not at zero risk. (15)

How does this information about the genetics of Alzheimer's disease apply to the case of Tom Morris and a decision about undergoing genetic testing? Given the age of onset of Alzheimer's disease for Tom's grandfather, father, and uncle, he has a family history of *late-onset* Alzheimer's disease, possibly related genetically to APOE e4. If Tom undergoes genetic testing for APOE e4 and tests positive, he learns only that he has an increased likelihood of developing late-onset Alzheimer's disease. This information would be useful to him if it could guide preventative care. In other words, having this information would be a strong argument in favor of Tom undergoing genetic testing if effective ways could be found (for example, through medication or life-style modifications) to delay or prevent the occurrence of late-onset Alzheimer's disease. (11) Thus the value of genetic testing for Tom interfaces with the larger medical issue of what is (or is not) available for treating Alzheimer's disease.

Genetic Discrimination

As already mentioned, individuals may be reluctant to undergo genetic testing because they fear that a positive test result may cause loss of employment or health insurance. In considering such "genetic discrimination" we will focus on the issue of health insurance.

There are a number of ways in which an insurance company might use genetic information. The company might use it to determine an applicant's eligibility for insurance. (17, 18) For example, in the case involving Tom Morris, a positive genetic test for APOE e4, which increases the likelihood of developing late-onset Alzheimer's disease, might disqualify him from obtaining long-term care insurance. (19) An insurance company might also use genetic information to set rates. On the one hand, a company might charge higher than standard rates to those genetically at risk for a disease. On the other hand, an insurer might "offer preferred policies to those people who voluntarily come forward with genetic information that indicates that they do not have any elevated risk" for a genetically based disease. (18) From a client's perspective, such practices may seem discriminatory. (20) For fear of such discrimination, some people might decide to forgo genetic testing that could be of benefit to them. (21)

A major line of argument in favor of prohibiting access to and use of genetic information by insurers is the fact that which genes each of us has is purely a matter of chance. No one has control over his or her genetic makeup as indicated by such terminology as "genetic lottery" and "genetic dice." (22) Since our genes are "not our fault," it is argued that it would not be fair to discriminate against individuals on the basis of their genetic makeup:

> The moral cornerstone of the criticism seems to be that it is wrong to use genetic information for discriminatory purposes because, from the moral point of view, those who have lost out in nature's genetic lottery do not deserve their bad fortune any more (or perhaps deserve it even less) than those who have been favored by the genetic dice deserve their good fortune. According to the critics, to discriminate against an individual on the basis of genetic test information would be to disadvantage them on the basis of purely accidental, morally irrelevant characteristics. (22)

On the other hand, private insurance companies might argue for having access to and using genetic information about clients on the basis of *actuarial fairness*. This is a claim that "fair treatment of persons requires classifying them according to their risks and making underwriting decisions—whether to offer a policy, with what terms, at what cost—in accordance with those risks." (18) Using the concept of actuarial fairness, "insurers claim they would be acting unjustly if they offered essentially the same terms and rates to persons with different risks." (18) Thus, if an individual's genetic makeup adversely affects his or her risk of disease or death, it is rightly taken into account by an insurance company. Indeed, from the perspective of the insurance company, "the more information which it can accumulate about a potential insured, the more accurate—in theory at least—will be its assessment of risk and the more appropriate will be the premium demanded." (23)

In evaluating this line of argument, one relevant question concerns the potential of genetic information to give accurate assessment of risks. It has been suggested that the "insurer's view that genetic information is important to accurately assess the future risk of an individual making a claim . . . perpetuates a deterministic view of disease" when in fact it is the case that "defining the clinical utility of a genetic test is a rather complex task." (20) In this regard it has been noted that

> . . . genetic tests can provide more accurate information about the subject's future health status only in the case of certain relatively simple single gene disorders, such as Huntington's disease and cystic fibrosis, [and] even in these cases the genetic tests are not considered to be completely foolproof. In more complex and, from the viewpoint of insurance companies, more interesting, disorders such as Alzheimer's disease and cancer, the predictive accuracy of the genetic test is considerably less, estimated to be of the same (or even lower) accuracy of prediction as standard non-genetic medical tests. (22)

Furthermore, some have raised questions about the appropriateness of using the principle of actuarial fairness (22):

> There is yet another possibility: that the central notion underlying commercial health insurance underwriting—the greater the likelihood of illness, the more one should pay for coverage—is morally unsound. (24)

Rather, it has been suggested that "health care, and the insurance that helps pay for it, ought to be available according to need. . . ." (18) This contention makes sense if one believes that everyone has a "right" to health care, or at least, to a certain basic level of health care. This contention also suggests thinking of insurance more on the model of a "public utility" rather than a private business. There is some evidence that we do, in fact, think this way. While "coverage through a private insurer may not be an entitlement, certainly the U.S.

population and government have agreed that medical care is an entitlement as evidenced by the Medicare and Medicaid systems. . . ." (12)

One approach that may be taken to the problem of genetic discrimination in health insurance (and in other areas) is legislative. In this regard, it is important to recognize that laws and governmental regulations must address the realm of *genetic information* in general as well as genetic testing. Otherwise, someone (such as Tom Morris) might be denied insurance simply on the basis of information about family history although the individual himself has not undergone personal genetic testing to determine if he has inherited the deleterious gene. (25) Indeed, he may in fact be free of it. Denying someone health insurance on such a basis does not seem to be just.

This chapter has focused on one genetically based disease, Alzheimer's disease. However, it should be kept in mind that every one of us "has some genetic predisposition, condition or disease resulting from inherited or acquired genetic changes." (26) Concomitantly, "since each individual carries a number of mutated genes, genetic discrimination . . . threaten[s] each of us." (26) For this reason, the presence or absence of legal protections in the use of genetic information is a matter of concern for all of us.

CHAPTER SUMMARY

Key Terms and Concepts

Human Genome Project (HGP): a scientific project identifying all the genes in human DNA and determining the sequences of the chemical base pairs that make up human DNA.
ELSI: a project studying ethical, legal, and social issues resulting from the Human Genome Project.
presymptomatic genetic testing: testing to determine if an individual carries a form of a gene related to the occurrence of a particular disease before the individual actually shows symptoms of the disease.
early-onset Alzheimer's disease: the symptoms of Alzheimer's disease start before the age of 55.
late-onset Alzheimer's disease: the symptoms of Alzheimer's disease occur after age 65.
actuarial fairness: a concept in the insurance industry claiming that fair treatment of persons requires classifying them according to their risks and making underwriting decisions in accordance with those risks.

Key Points

- In considering the ethical, legal, and social implications of current work in the field of genetics, four areas have been identified as requiring discussion and reflection among health care professionals and patients: privacy and fair use of genetic information; responsible clinical integration of genetic information; stigmatization and discrimination based on genetic traits; and professional and public education.
- Benefits of presymptomatic genetic testing include a sense of relief from the uncertainty of not knowing one's genetic status, the opportunity to make plans for the future in the event of a positive test result, and, in some cases, the opportunity to take steps to prevent or delay the onset of symptoms of the disease.
- Harmful consequences of presymptomatic genetic testing may include a negative psychological impact of a positive test result, experiencing genetic discrimination (e.g., in employment and health insurance), a sense of guilt over the possibility of having transmitted the genetic disorder to one's children, and a feeling of guilt on the part of individuals who have tested negative while other family members have tested positive.
- An argument in favor of health insurers having access to and using genetic information is based on the concept of actuarial fairness, which classifies persons according to their risks and makes underwriting decisions in accordance with those risks.
- A major line of argument in support of prohibiting access to and use of genetic information by health insurers is the fact that which genes each of us has is purely a matter of chance. Further, it is argued that health care, and the insurance that helps pay for it, ought to be available according to need.
- Effective legal protections against genetic discrimination must cover genetic information in general, and not be limited to genetic testing.

FOR FURTHER DISCUSSION

1. In the case study at the beginning of this chapter, Tom Morris is engaged to be married. Do you think that he has an ethical obligation to his future spouse to undergo genetic testing for late-onset Alzheimer's disease and to share the test results with her before they marry?
2. Suppose that Tom Morris had a family history of early-onset Alzheimer's disease. In this case, do you think that Tom has an ethical obligation to his

future spouse to undergo genetic testing for Alzheimer's and to share the test results with her before they marry? Or, from an ethical point of view, is it enough if Tom's future spouse is simply aware of the family history of early-onset Alzheimer's disease?

3. Tom Morris has two older sisters who are likewise at risk of having inherited the gene variant for late-onset Alzheimer's disease. His sisters may or may not be aware of a genetic basis for this condition. From an ethical point of view, should Tom warn his sisters that they are at risk and that genetic testing is available? Would your judgment be different if the family history involved early-onset Alzheimer's disease?

4. Has anyone in your family (or a close acquaintance) undergone genetic testing? How was the testing handled? Did the person ever regret undergoing genetic testing?

5. Has anyone in your family (or a close acquaintance) been affected by a genetic disease? Has that person ever experienced any discrimination, with respect to employment or insurance or otherwise?

6. Because of the potential for genetic discrimination, someone may wish to undergo genetic testing to find out information that is personally valuable but not want the fact of the genetic testing or the results to be included in his or her medical record. From an ethical point of view, do you think such a request should be honored? Explain your response.

References

1. U.S. Department of Energy, *Human Genome Project Information.* http://www.ornl.gov/sci/techresources/Human_Genome/home.shtml. Accessed May 2009.
2. Catholic Health Association of the United States, *Facilitator's Resource Manual for Harnessing the Promise of Genomics* (St. Louis, MO: Catholic Health Association of the United States, 2004).
3. C.A. Christianson, K.M. McWalter, and N.S. Warren, "Assessment of allied health graduates' preparation to integrate genetic knowledge and skills into clinical practice," *Journal of Allied Health* 34/3 (Fall 2005): 138-44.
4. J.H. Marks and M.L. Richter, "The genetic associate: a new health professional," *American Journal of Public Health* 66/4 (1976): 388-90.
5. T.R. Mertens, J.R. Hendrix, K.M. Kenkel, "The genetic associate: a career option in genetic counseling," *The Journal of Heredity* 77/3 (May-June 1986): 175-78.

6. Ricki Lewis, *Human Genetics Concepts and Applications,* 5th ed. (New York: McGraw-Hill, 2003).
7. *Do You Really Want to Know?* CBS 60 Minutes. Video.
8. U.S. Department of Energy, *Human Genome Project Information: Ethical, Legal & Social Issues.* http://www.ornl.gov/sci/techresources/Human_Genome/elsi/esli.html. Accessed May 2009.
9. Michael Smith, Jerome V. Danoff, Mina Jain, and Toby M. Long, "Genetic Disorders: Implications for Allied Health Professionals Two Case Studies," *Internet Journal of Allied Health Sciences and Practice* 5/4 (Oct. 2007). http://ijahsp.nova.edu/articles/vol5num4/pdf/danoff.pdf. Accessed May 2009.
10. Jean F. Jenkins and Dale Halsey Lea, *Nursing Care in the Genomic Era A Case-Based Approach* (Boston: Jones and Bartlett, 2005).
11. National Institute on Aging of the National Institutes of Health, *Alzheimer's Disease Genetics Fact Sheet* (Nov. 2008; updated May 2009). http://www.nia.nih.gov/Alzheimers/Publications/geneticsfs.htm. Accessed May 2009.
12. Mignon Fogarty, "Genetic Testing, Alzheimer Disease, and Long-Term Care Insurance," *Genetic Testing* 3/1 (1999): 133-37.
13. Robert Mullan Cook-Deegan, "Some Questions Arising in the Commercial Development of Genetic Tests for Alzheimer Disease" in Stephen G. Post and Peter J. Whitehouse (eds.), *Genetic Testing for Alzheimer Disease Ethical and Clinical Issues* (Baltimore: Johns Hopkins University Press, 1998).
14. Peter H. St. George-Hyslop, "Molecular Genetics of Early-Onset Alzheimer Disease Linked to Chromosome 14 and Chromosome 21" in Stephen G. Post and Peter J. Whitehouse (eds.), *Genetic Testing for Alzheimer Disease Ethical and Clinical Issues* (Baltimore: Johns Hopkins University Press, 1998).
15. Kimberly A. Quaid, "Implications of Genetic Susceptibility Testing with Apolipoprotein E," in Stephen G. Post and Peter J. Whitehouse (eds.), *Genetic Testing for Alzheimer Disease Ethical and Clinical Issues* (Baltimore: Johns Hopkins University Press, 1998).
16. Stephen G. Post, Peter J. Whitehouse, and Arthur B. Zinn, "Introduction Genetics and the Moral Future of Dementia Care" in Stephen G. Post and Peter J. Whitehouse (eds.), *Genetic Testing for Alzheimer Disease Ethical and Clinical Issues* (Baltimore: Johns Hopkins University Press, 1998).
17. Nancy E. Kass, "Insurance for the Insurers The Use of Genetic Tests," *Hastings Center Report* 22/6 (Nov./Dec. 1992): 6-11.
18. Robert H. Binstock and Thomas H. Murray, "Genetics and Long-Term-Care Insurance," in Stephen G. Post and Peter J. Whitehouse (eds.), *Genetic Testing for Alzheimer Disease Ethical and Clinical Issues* (Baltimore: Johns Hopkins University Press, 1998).

19. American Geriatrics Society Ethics Committee, Position Statement, *Genetic Testing for Late-Onset Alzheimer's Disease* (Nov. 2000). http://www.americangeriatrics.org/products/ positionpapers/gen test.shtml. Accessed May 2009.
20. Elias Mossialos and Anna Dixon, "Genetic Testing and insurance: opportunities and challenges for society," *Trends in Molecular Medicine* 7/7 (July 2001): 323-24.
21. E. David Cook, "Genetics and the British insurance industry," *Journal of Medical Ethics* 25 (1999): 157-62.
22. Veikko Launis, "The Use of Genetic Test Information in Insurance: The Argument from Indistinguishability Reconsidered," *Science and Engineering Ethics* 6 (2000): 299-310.
23. Sheila A.M. McLean and Philippa Gannon, "Genetics and Insurance" in Tom Sorell (ed.), *Health Care, Ethics and Insurance* (New York: Routledge, 1998).
24. Thomas H. Murray, "Genetics and the Moral Mission of Health Insurance," *Hastings Center Report* 22/6 (Nov./Dec. 1992): 12-17.
25. Tony Leys, "Daily Fear: Will Curse Strike?" *Des Moines Register* (August 21, 2001): 1A, 5A.
26. Genetic Alliance, *Genetic Discrimination in Health Insurance and Employment Act.* http://www.geneticalliance.org/geneticissues/gainsurance.html. Accessed 2003.

Index

abortion
  brain activity, 36–37
  case studies, 32–33, 39–40
  controversy, compared to euthanasia controversy, 73
  cultural differences, 19
  direct vs. indirect, 31–32
  effects upon marriage, 32–34
  ethics and, 16–18
  "human being vs. human person" debate, 38–40
  induced or procured, 31
  preimplantation genetic diagnosis and, 42–43
  rape, 43–44
  reasons for and against, 33–34
  relativism vs. objectivism, 19
  selective, 40–43
  twinning and fusion of embryos, 37
  wastage, natural, 37–38
abuse, child
  families with disabled children, 68
  government's role as *parens patriae*, 72–73, 195
accommodations, multicultural, 208
acquired immune deficiency syndrome (AIDS) and confidentiality, 169
actuarial fairness and genetics, 265–66
act-utilitarianism, 9–10
addiction, defined, 156
adoption vs. artificial insemination by donor (AID), 52

advance directives. *See also* durable power of attorney for health care; living will
  advantages, 105–6
  competence, mental, 102–3
  documentation, 107
  vs. do-not-resuscitate (DNR) orders, 107
  durable power of attorney for health care, 101–2
  education, 105
  executing, 102–4
  Five Wishes, 107–8
  language, nonspecific, 106
  living will, 101–2
  objections of conscience, 197
  Patient Self-Determination Act, 104–5, 197
  POLST (Physician Orders for Life-Sustaining Treatment) Paradigm Initiative, 108
  problems, 106–7
allocation
  donated organs, 249–53
  staff time and services, 181–83
altruistic donation of organs and tissues, 246–48
Alzheimer's disease
  case study, 149–50
  genetic testing, 263–64
  stem cell research, 236
American Bar Association, Commission on Legal Problems of the Elderly, 103
American Diabetic Association (ADA)
  Ethical and Legal Issues in Nutrition, Hydration, and Feeding, 123–24

guidelines for patients in vegetative states, 141
Issues in Feeding the Terminally Ill Adult, 122–23
position on assisted nutrition and hydration, 116
American Hospital Association Special Committee on Biomedical Ethics, 197
American Medical Association (AMA) Council on Ethical and Judicial Affairs, 69, 91–92, 158
anencephaly, 65, 134
antibiotics
   end-of-life directives, 108
   palliative care, 86
   viral vs. bacterial pneumonia, 85
Aquinas, Thomas, 14
Arenella, Dr. Cheryl, 118
artificial insemination (AI), 51
artificial insemination by donor (AID)
   vs. adoption, 52
   arguments for and against, 51–53
   Canadian study, 52
   case study, 50
   psychological effects, 52–53
artificial insemination by husband (AIH), 51
assistance for families with disabled children, 68
assisted nutrition and hydration
   advance directives, 108
   American Diabetic Association guidelines, 116, 141
   benefits and burdens, weighing, 117–19, 136–38
   Catholic church, position on, 116–17
   dehydration, effects of, 120–21
   Ethical and Legal Issues in Nutrition, Hydration, and Feeding (American Diabetic Association), 123–24
   Issues in Feeding the Terminally Ill Adult (American Diabetic Association), 122–23
   medical treatment vs. standard care, 115–17
   misunderstandings, common, 120–22
assisted reproductive technologies (ART)
   artificial insemination by donor (AID), 51–53
   case study, 50
   in vitro fertilization (IVF), 57–59
   surrogacy, 54–56
assisted suicide. *See also* euthanasia
   arguments for and against, 150–55
   case study, 148–50
   ethics, 15
autonomy of patient. *See also* durable power of attorney for health care
   attention to, 183–84
   confidentiality, 168
   emphasis on, in Western culture, 205–6, 208–9
   free and informed consent, 224–27
   In re Brooks Estate, 193–94
   life-sustaining treatments, 83–85
   organ donation, 247–48
   Patient Self-Determination Act, 104–5, 197
   principle of, 4–8
   proxy for patient in vegetative state, 137
   refusal of treatment on religious grounds, 193–96
   terminal illness, 205–8

balance of harm and benefit, and medical research, 222
Beauchamp, Tom, 4
Beckwith-Wiedemann syndrome, 57
Belmont Report, 218
beneficence, principle of, 4–8, 180, 194, 222
benefits and burdens, weighing
   assisted nutrition and dehydration, 122–23
   care, palliative, 119–19
   consciousness, 84, 136–38
   financial resources, 86, 140
   life-sustaining treatments, 83–85, 118–19
   pain management, 84
   patients in vegetative states, 136–38
   patient's perspective, 85
   quality of life, 85
   research, medical, with human subjects, 222
Bentham, Jeremy, 8–10
best interests standard, 69–73, 100–1
bio-ethical issues, presidential commission on, 140

biological family ties and artificial insemination by donor (AID), 52
biological life vs. mental activities, 139–40
birth defects
    issues regarding, in surrogate birth, 55
    occurrence of, in IVF process, 57
blood transfusion
    case study, 192
    In re Brooks Estate, 193–94
    Jehovah's Witnesses, religious objection, 193–96
    pregnant mother, 195
brain activity
    criteria for determining degree of unconsciousness, 133–34
    determining death, 36–37
    vegetative states, 133–34, 139–40
brain death, 36–37, 244–46
brain injury, 135. *See also* vegetative states, patient in
brain stem, 133
Brooks, Bernice, 193–94
Buddhism, preference for clarity of mind at death, 209–10

Callahan, Daniel, 87
Canadian study of artificial insemination by donor (AID), 52
cardiac death, controlled donation after, 245–46
"care, not cure" slogan, 88
care, comfort
    dehydration, effects and benefits of, 121
    Five Wishes document, 108–9
    nonmedical means of, 108
    personal vs. impersonal nutrition and hydration, 121–22
care, palliative. *See also* death and dying
    benefits and burdens of life-sustaining treatments, 118–19
    case for better, in contrast with euthanasia, 155–59
    hospice, 118–19, 121
    Kübler-Ross, Elizabeth, 206
    organ donation, 246
    sedation, terminal, 158–59
    use of antibiotics, 86

care, standard health
    assisted nutrition and hydration, 116–18, 121–22
    vs. medical treatment, 115–17
case studies
    amniocentesis and decision making, 39–40
    artificial insemination by donor (AID), 50
    assisted suicide and euthanasia, 148–50
    chemotherapy, ending treatment, 82–83
    confidentiality, 168
    do-not-resuscitate (DNS) order, 88–89
    genetics, 260
    newborn, seriously ill, 66–67
    objection of conscience, 196
    objection, religious, to blood transfusion, 192
    obligations of health care professionals, 180–81, 183–85
    organ donation, 244, 248
    patient in vegetative state, 132–33
    research and experimentation with human subjects, 219
    recipient of donated organs, 248
    stem cell research, 234
    twins, in surrogate birth, 53–54
categorical imperative, Kant's, 10–12
Catholic Church
    Ethical and Religious Directives for Catholic Health Care Services, 205–6
    position on assisted nutrition and hydration, 116–17
Center for Ethics in Health Care, 108
children
    best interests of, 69–71
    consensus, in care decisions for elder, 8
    divorce, in families with disabled children, 68
    parens patriae power of government, 72–73, 195
    risks to, caused by in vitro fertilization, 57
    sibling relationships, 55–56
    welfare of, and surrogacy, 55–56
Childress, James, 4
Cicero, 14
clinical integration of genetic information, 261–62

cloning (somatic cell nuclear transfer), 237–39
codes of research ethics, 218
coma. *See also* vegetative state, patient in
  American Diabetic Association (ADA) guidelines, 141
  defined, 135
  "human being vs. human person" debate, 38–40
comfort care. *See* care, comfort
Commission on Legal Problems of the Elderly, 103
committee, ethics, 26–27
communication
  ethics committees, 27
  multicultural needs, 208
  patient's ability, 84, 133
  truth-telling vs. lying, 205–8
communitarian view on organ donation, 247
compassion, 150
compensation, financial incentives for organs, 246–47
competence, mental
  advance directives, 102–3, 107
  assisted nutrition and dehydration, 123
  consent, proxy, 227–28
  refusal of treatment on religious grounds, 194–95
conception/fertilization
  abortion debate, 35–36
  beginning of life, 43
confidentiality
  autonomy of patient, 168
  breaking, 169–70
  case study, 168
  disclosure by patients, 168–69
  Hippocratic oath, 167
  job descriptions of health care providers, 171–72
  utilitarian ethics, 9–10
conflict resolution, 208
consciousness. *See also* unconsciousness
  Buddhist preference for clarity of mind at death, 209–10
  locked-in syndrome, 135
  minimally conscious state, 135
  newborn, seriously ill or disabled, 69, 134
  weighing benefits and burdens of treatments, 84, 136–38
consensus, in decision making, 8
consent
  free and informed, 224–27, 235
  IRB worksheet, 220–21, 226
  multicultural views on, 210–11
  presumed, in organ donation, 247–48
  proxy, for medical research, 227–28
  stem cell research, 235
consequentialist ethical theories, 8–10, 169
consultations
  ethics, 27–28
  case by case, 26
contribution, principle of, 5, 181
controlled donation after cardiac death, 245
controversy
  abortion vs. euthanasia, 73
  cloning, 237–39
  homosexuality, 17
  newborns, seriously ill, 65–74
  somatic cell nuclear transfer (SCNT), 237–39
  stem cell research, 236–39
Council on Ethical and Judicial Affairs, 158
counseling for families with disabled children, 68
court cases, 193–194
cranial-nerve reflexes, 134
Cruzan, Nancy, 104, 113, 116, 131
Curren, Judith, 155
cultural relativism, 18
cystic fibrosis, case study, 39–40

dead donor rule, 244
death and dying. *See also* assisted suicide; care, palliative; euthanasia
  assisted nutrition and hydration, 120–22
  conscious patient, 101
  criteria for determining, 244–45
  determining, and abortion debate, 36–37
  with dignity, 151
  fear of process of, 155
  hospice, 118–19, 121
  Kübler-Ross, Elizabeth, 206
  living will, 101–2
  medical interventions, defined, 90–91

multicultural views on pain management, 209–10
newborn, seriously ill or disabled, 69–70, 134
organ donation, 244–46
palliative care, 88, 155–59, 246
truth-telling to the terminally ill, 205–8
"whole brain death," 244
withdrawing treatment vs. euthanasia, 87, 198
Deatherage-Newsome, Blaine, 41–42
Debringer, Dr. Konrad, 194
decision making
ethics committees, 25–28
health-care proxy, and difficulty "letting go," 107
life-sustaining treatments, 83–86
patients in vegetative states, 136–40
process for determining futility of treatment, 91–92
rights of parents, 72
standards for treatment of seriously ill newborns, 69–73
substituted judgment, 100–1, 137
Declaration of Helsinki, 218
dehydration, effects of, 120–21. See also assisted nutrition and hydration
Demange, Dr. Gilbert, 194
dependence, drug, 156
diagnosis, lethal
"letting die" vs. "killing," 88
medical futility, 90
truth-telling to terminally ill patients, 205–8
dietitians, role in assisted nutrition and hydration, 124
dignity, human, 151
directed versus nondirected organ donation, 249
directives, advance. See advance directives
disabilities
newborns, seriously ill, 65–74, 134
quality of life and, 41–42, 67–68
disabled vs. dying, 138–40
disclosure, confidentiality and, 168–69
discrimination
genetic traits, 262, 265–67
organ donation, 250

disease, genetic, preimplantation diagnosis, 42–43
disease, incurable or irreversible
living will, 101–2
truth-telling to terminally ill patients, 205-8
disease, infectious, and health care providers' responsibilities, 179–80
divorce, in families with disabled children, 68
Dolly (cloned sheep), 238
do-not-resuscitate (DNR) orders, 107
donors
altruistic donation, 246
national donor registry, 248
organ, 246–48
recipients of organs, 249–53
sperm, 53
waiting list exchange, 249
double effect, principle of, 15–16, 156–57
Down syndrome, 41, 70–71
durable power of attorney for health care. See also advance directives; living will
appointing, 101–2
assisted nutrition and dehydration, 123
conscience clause, in Patient Self-Determination Act, 197
problems with, 107
vs. power of attorney, 102

economic issues, 55
education
advance directives, 105
ethics, and committees, 26
genetics, 262
effort, principle of, 5
elders, care of, 8. See also advance directives; death and dying
embryos and fetuses. See also pregnancy
abnormalities, selective abortion for, 40–42
beginnings of life, 35–38
"human being" vs. "human person" debate, 38–40
in vitro fertilization (IVF), 57–58
multifetal pregnancy, 2, 57
"spare," in in vitro fertilization, 57–58
stem cell research, 235–237
twinning, fusion, and natural wastage, 37

emotional issues. *See also* psychological issues
  advance directives, 107
  forgoing life-sustaining treatment, 84, 107, 198
  genetic testing, 263
  effects of seriously ill newborns on family, 67–68
emotional states of vegetative patients, 139
employment difficulties
  families with disabled children, 68
  genetic testing, 263, 265–67
end in itself principle (Kant), 11
end-of-life directives. *See* advance directives
equality, principle of, 5, 181
Ethical and Legal Issues in Nutrition, Hydration, and Feeding (American Diabetic Association), 123–24
Ethical and Religious Directives for Catholic Health Care Services, 205–6
ethical egoist, 8
ethical, legal, and social implications (ELSI) of genetics, 261–62
ethical relativism vs. ethical objectivism, 210–11
ethics. *See also* principles; rights; standards of care (feminist theory), 7–8
  consequentialist, 8–10
  contribution, 5
  defined, 1
  dilemmas, 6–7
  education on, and committees, 26
  of health care, 2–3
  individual patients, care of, 3
  inquiry, two levels of, 3
  justice, distributive, 6
  Kant's categorical imperative, 10–12
  nonmaleficence, 4–5
  "nothing is lost" principle, 237
  objectivism, 17–20
  organizational, of health care facility, 3
  principles, four basic, 4–8
  professionals in, 2–3
  relativism vs. objectivism, 17–20, 210–11
  rights-based, 12–14
  stem cell research, 236–39
  theories of, 3–20
Ethics and Social Impact Committee, 252

ethics committee
  determining futility of medical treatment, 91–92
  role in assisted nutrition and hydration, 124
ethnocentrism, defined, 17
eugenics program, 53
euthanasia. *See also* assisted suicide
  arguments for and against, 150–55
  case study, 148–50
  common misunderstandings, 120–22
  ethics and, 15
  financial resources, 153–54
  Groningen Protocol, 74–75
  involuntary, 147–48, 154–55
  life expectancy and, 152
  vs. life-sustaining treatment, 73–74
  living will, 101–2
  Netherlands, the, 148, 154–55
  palliative care, in contrast with, 155–59
  parenting, and informed consent to, 74
  physician-assisted suicide, 148
  quality of life and, 152
  seriously ill and disabled newborns, 73–74
  society and, 155
  utilitarianism, and assisted suicide, 11–12, 152
  voluntary vs. involuntary, 147–48, 154–55
  vs. withdrawing treatment, 87, 198
exercises, for patient in vegetative state, 136

facilities, long-term care, and health-care proxy, 107
Fairfax Cryobank (Virginia), 53
faith-healing services, 196
family. *See also* genetics
  advance directives, 105–6
  assistance for, with disabled children, 68
  effects on, of seriously ill newborns, 67–68
  effects on, of surrogacy, 55–56
  Hastings Center studies, 42, 67–68, 74
  involuntary euthanasia, 148
  involvement, multicultural views, 209
  Latino family-oriented views on health care, 209
  litigation and advance directives, 105–6
  medical history, 52, 262–67

naming of proxy decision maker, 107
organ donation, 246, 247
palliative care, 88
quality of life, with disabled/seriously ill children, 42
surrogacy, and relationship of parent and child, 55
withholding vs. withdrawing life-sustaining treatment, 87
feeding. *See* total parenteral feeding; intravenous feeding, central; peripheral intravenous feeding, 113, tube feeding
feminism
   concern for children, 55
   ethics of care, 7–8
   reproductive rights of women, 33–34
   surrogacy, views on, 55
fertility drugs and procedures. *See also* assisted reproductive technologies
   ethical issues raised by, 2
   in vitro fertilization, 57
fetus. *See* embryos and fetuses.
financial incentives for organs, 246–47
financial resources
   argument against assisted suicide and euthanasia, 153–54
   elder care, 86
   operation of health care facility, 3
   society and euthanasia, 155
   weighing benefits and burdens, 86, 140
First Amendment right, in *In re Brooks Estate*, 193–94
Five Wishes document, 108
Forbes, Chuck, 56
futility, medical, 89–91

gastrostomy tube, 114, 136
gastrulation, and abortion debate, 37
genetics. *See also* family
   case study, 260
   continuity, 52–53
   discrimination, 265–67
   ethical, legal, and social implications (ELSI), 261–62
   eugenics program, 53
   "genetic lottery" or "genetic dice," 265
   Human Genome Project (259–60)

preimplantation diagnosis, in IVF, 42–43
surrogacy, and relationship of parent and child, 55
therapeutic donor insemination (TDI), 51
"Georgetown mantra," of four principles, 4
goals of patient and family, 90
"golden rule," 10
Good Samaritan parable, 43–44
"greatest good for the greatest number," 8
Groningen Protocol, 74–75
guardian, court-appointed
   advance directives, 103
   parens patriae, government role as, 72–73, 195
   refusal of treatment on religious grounds, 195
guidelines
   American Diabetic Association, and patients' rights, 141
   ethics committees and, 26
   patients in vegetative states, 141
Hastings Center
   families with seriously ill or disabled children, 42
   study on imperiled newborns, 67–68, 74
health care
   China's views on, 210–11
   at home, for seriously ill newborns, 67
   standards for treatment decision making, 69–71
health care professionals (HCPs)
   advance (end-of-life) directives, 108
   case study, 180–81, 183–85
   confidentiality, exceptional cases, 170
   creative scheduling, 183
   job descriptions, 171–72
   litigation and advance directives, 105–6
   objections of conscience, 197–99
   obligations to provide care, 179–80
   personal obligations, 179–80
   primary image of, 155
   problems with co-workers, 185–86
   SARS outbreak, 179–80
   training in pain management, 156
   training in privacy practices, 172
   using own judgment, 183–84

health care services
  allocation of staff time and services, 181–83
  objections to care, 193–99
health insurance. *See* insurance, health
Health Insurance Portability and Accountability Act (HIPAA) regulations, 6, 172–73
Hippocratic oath of confidentiality, 167
HIV (human immunodeficiency virus)
  assisted nutrition, 118
  breaking confidentiality, 170
Hobbes, Thomas, 14
homosexuality, controversy of, 17
hope, false, 89
hospice. *See also* care, palliative
  benefits and burdens of palliative care, 118–19
  dehydration, effects of, 121
  Kübler-Ross, Elizabeth, 206
Human Genome Project (HGP), 259–60
human subjects
  notorious experiments, 217–18
  Institutional Review Board worksheet, 220–21
human wholeness
  refusal of treatment on religious grounds, 194
  vegetative states of patients, 139–40
hyperalimentation, 114
hypothalamus, 133

illness, mental, 169. *See also* competence, mental
illness, terminal, and disclosing, 205–8, 210–11
imperative, categorical (Kant), 10–13
In re Brooks Estate, 193–94
insemination. *See* artificial insemination (AI); artificial insemination by donor (AID)
intravenous feeding, central, 114. *See also* total parenteral feeding; tube feeding
incontinence, 134
induced pluripotent stem cells, 235
infertility
  assisted reproductive technologies, 49–59
  male, causes of, 51

informed consent, in medical research, 222, 224–27
immune rejection, 235
in-service programs, 26
Institutional Review Board (IRB)
  funding from U.S. Department of Health and Human Services, 218
  worksheet, 220–221
insurance, health
  Health Insurance Portability and Accountability Act (HIPAA) regulations, 6, 172–73
  Medicare and/or Medicaid, 104–5, 267
  preventing discrimination based on genetic traits, 262–63, 265–67
investigators, in medical research, 222
in vitro fertilization (IVF)
  abortion, 42–43
  embryonic stem cell research, 235
  ethics, 15, 57
  "spare" fetuses, 57–58
Issues in Feeding the Terminally Ill Adult (American Diabetic Association), 122–23

Jehovah's Witnesses, 193–95
jejunostomy tube, 114, 136
John Paul II, Pope, 116–17
justice, distributive, 4–6, 13, 181, 222, 251–52
justice-over-a-lifetime, in organ donation, 252

Kant, Immanuel, 10–12
Kantian ethics
  assisted reproductive technologies, 58
  categorical imperative, 10–12
  persons, respecting, 11–12, 222
  surrogacy, 56
Kennedy Institute of Ethics at Georgetown University, 4
Kevorkian, Dr. Jack, 154–55
killing
  general prohibition against, 152
  vs. "letting die," 87
Kübler-Ross, Elizabeth, 206

Lauritzen, Paul, 58
law
  end in itself (Kant), 11

natural, 14–16, 152
universal (Kant), 11
life. *See also* quality of life
   beginnings of, 34–40
   biological, 139–40
   expectancy, 152–53
   preimplantation genetic diagnosis and, 42–43
   viability of fetus, 35
life-sustaining treatments. *See also* nutrition and hydration, assisted
   advance directives, 106–7
   benefits vs. burdens, weighing, 83–85
   case studies, 82–83, 86–88
   court cases, well-known, 104
   forgoing, 86–89, 106–7, 124, 135–38, 198
   "heroic," 124
   living will, 101–2
   medical risks, 118–19
   misconceptions about forgoing, 86–89
   organ donation, 245
   POLST (Physician Orders for Life-Sustaining Treatment) Paradigm Initiative, 108
   vegetative states and decision making, 136–40
   withholding vs. withdrawing, 86–88
living will, 101–2. *See also* advance directives; durable power of attorney for health care
   assisted nutrition and dehydration, 123
   conscience clause, in Patient Self-Determination Act, 197
Locke, John, 14
locked-in syndrome, 135
love, as necessary in palliative care, 159

malnutrition. *See* nutrition and hydration, assisted
mandated choice, for organ donation, 248
marriage
   abortion debate, 32–34
   artificial insemination by donor (AID), 51–52
   infertility, 49–59
   infidelity, feelings of, 51
Medecins Sans Frontiers, 179–80
medical history of family, 52–53

medical indications policy standard, 69–71
medical interventions, futile or not, 90–91
medical professionals. *See* health care professionals (HCPs)
medical records
   confidentiality, 3, 168–72
   Health Insurance Portability and Accountability Act (HIPAA), 172–73
   Medicare and/or Medicaid advance directives, 104–5
   right to health care, 267
medication, pain, 155–59. *See also* pain and pain management
memory, in vegetative states, 139
Mill, John Stuart, 8–10
moral principles, 20, 252–53, 265–66. *See also* ethics
motherhood
   and abortion debate, 32–34
   surrogate, 8–9, 11, 35, 39
multicultural views
   Arab emphasis on "verbal" vs. "written" agreements, 210
   China's views on health care, 210–11
   individualism, stress on, in Western culture, 208–10
   Latino family-oriented views, 209
   relativism vs. objectivism, 16–20
   truth-telling to the terminally ill, 205–8
multifetal pregnancy
   in in vitro fertilization, 57
   McCaughey septuplets, 2

nasogastric (NG) tube, 114, 136
National Adult Literacy Survey (1993), 225
national donor registry, 248
natural law theory, 14–15
natural wastage, and abortion debate, 37–38
Nazi Germany and medical research, 217
need, principle of, 6, 181
negligence, 5–6
Netherlands, the, and euthanasia, 148, 154–55
newborns, seriously ill
   case study, 66–67
   controversy of, 65–74

Hastings Center study of effect on family, 67–68
standards for treatment decision making, 69–73
states of unconsciousness, 134
nonmaleficence, principle of
    children and effects of surrogacy, 56
    in vitro fertilization, 57
    multicultural views on, 211
    principle of, 4–5, 185
    research with human subjects, 222
Nuremberg Code, 218
nutrition and hydration, assisted. *See* assisted nutrition and hydration

objections of conscience, 197–99
Oregon Health and Sciences University, 108
organ donation
    allocating to recipients, 249–53
    case studies, 244, 248
    consent, presumed, 247–48
    controlled donation after cardiac death, 245
    dead donor rule, 244
    determining death, 244–46
    donors, recruiting, 246–48
    justice-over-a-lifetime, in allocation decisions, 252
    national donor registry, 248
    required response or mandated choice, 248
organizational ethics and ethics committees, 25
Outka, Gene H., 237
ovarian hyperstimulation syndrome (OHSS), 239

pain and pain management. *See also* life-sustaining treatments
    Buddhist views on end of life, 209–10
    lack of, in vegetative states, 135
    medication, in death and dying, 155–59
    reason for assisted suicide and euthanasia, 150
    reflex vs. conscious experience of, 135
    weighing benefits and burdens, 84
paired donation or paired exchange, in organ donation, 249

palliative care, 88
parens patriae power
    newborn, seriously ill, and, 72–73
    refusal of health care on religious grounds, 195
parenting
    abortion debate, 31–44
    best interest of the child, 69–71
    biological vs. gestational vs. social, 59
    challenges of, with seriously ill newborns, 67–68
    decision making, in cases of seriously ill newborns, 72
    difficulties of caretaking seriously ill newborns, 67–68
    disabled or ill children, 41–42, 68–73
    effects of assisted reproductive technologies, 52–53, 58–59
    government's role as *parens patriae*, 72–73, 195
    informed consent, for euthanasia, 74
    newborn, seriously ill, and, 70–73
    questions raised by artificial insemination, 52–53
    refusing treatment for child on religious grounds, 195–96
    relational potential standard, 69, 71
    selective abortion, 40–42
    single or same-sex, 53
Parkinson's disease, and stem cell research, 236
pastoral care and advance directives, 103
patient autonomy. *See* autonomy of patient
Patient Self-Determination Act, 104–5, 197
patients
    and proxy (surrogate) decision maker, 100–1, 137
    autonomy of, 83–86, 151, 205–8
    perspective, in weighing benefits and burdens, 85
peripheral intravenous feeding, 113
persistent vegetative state (PVS), 134–35
person, whole
    free and informed consent, 224–27
    refusal of treatment on religious grounds, 194
    respect for, 11–12, 222

See also Kantian ethics
vegetative states of patients, 139–40
personality, 139
physician-assisted suicide, 148. *See also* assisted suicide; euthanasia
physician's orders, assisted nutrition and hydration, 116
pneumonia, 85
policies and guidelines, ethics committees and, 26
POLST (Physician Orders for Life-Sustaining Treatment) Paradigm Initiative, 108
post-coma unresponsive. *See* vegetative state, patient in
power of attorney. *See* durable power of attorney for health care
pregnancy
   abortion debate, 31–44
   beginning stages of life and, 35–37
   multifetal, in in vitro fertilization, 57
   Roe v. Wade (1973), 35
preimplantation genetic diagnosis, 42–43
prejudice, and organ donation, 250
President's Commission for the Study of Ethical Problems in Medicine and Biomedical and Behavioral Research, 69
presumed consent, in organ donation, 247
presymptomatic genetic testing, 262–64
preventive care, for patient in vegetative state, 136
principles. *See also* ethics; rights; standards
   autonomy of patient, 83–85, 137, 205–8
   beneficence, 4–8, 180, 194
   benefits and burdens, weighing, 69, 83–86, 117–19, 136–38
   China's views on health care, 210–11
   confidentiality, 169–70
   contribution, 5, 181
   double effect, 156–57
   effort, 5
   equality, 5, 181
   justice, distributed, 5–6, 13, 181, 222, 251–52
   life-sustaining treatment, 83–86
   need, 5, 182
   nonmaleficence, 211
   objections, religious and ethical, to treatment, 193–99
   overview, 5
   respect for person, 11–12
   substituted judgment, 100–1, 137
Principles of Biomedical Ethics (Beauchamp and Childress), 4
privacy and fair use of genetic information, 261
Privacy Rule, Health Insurance Portability and Accountability Act (HIPAA), 172–73
pro-life advocates, 41
professional-patient relationship, confidentiality, 168–69
progress vs. cultural relativism, 18
prostitution
   ethics and, 12
   surrogacy, compared to, 55
proxy, health care. *See also* durable power of attorney for health care
   Five Wishes document, 109
   role in determining treatment, 91–92
   substituted judgment, 100–1, 137
psychological issues. *See also* emotional issues
   benefits and burdens, weighing, 84
   child of assisted reproduction, 58–59
   child, unplanned, 34
   effects of forcing treatment, 194
   family, in artificial insemination by donor (AID), 52
   multicultural views on "truth-telling," 207–8
   proxy for health care and difficulty "letting go," 107
   siblings, in surrogate births, 55–56
   terminally ill patients and truth-telling, 205–8
   women choosing abortion, 34
   withholding vs. withdrawing life-sustaining treatment, 87

quality of life. *See also* life
   assisted suicide and euthanasia, 152
   benefits and burdens, weighing, 85
   families with disabled children, 41–42, 68–73
   futility of medical intervention, 90–91
Quinlan, Karen Ann, 104, 131

rape, abortion and, 43–44
records, medical. 3, 168–73
regulations, federal, and informed consent, 224–25
relationships, 69, 71, 168–69. *See also* family
relativism vs. objectivism, 19
religious views
    abortion and, 43–44
    Jehovah's Witnesses and refusal of blood transfusions, 193–96
    Catholic position on assisted nutrition and hydration, 116–17
    objections to health care practices, 193–96
Repository for Germinal Choice, 53
    reproductive rights, 33–34
reproductive technologies. *See* assisted reproductive technologies (ART)
required response, for organ donation, 248
research, medical
    breakthroughs, 153
    design, good, 222
    experiments with human subjects, notorious, 217–18
    Institutional Review Board (IRB), sample worksheet, 220–22
    norms and principles regarding, 222–23
    stem cell, 235–39
    subjects in institutional settings, 223
    therapeutic vs. nontherapeutic, 227–28
resources, allocation of
    health care professionals' time and services, 181–83
    patients in vegetative states, 139
respiration, depression of, 156–57
resuscitation, and advance directives, 108. *See also* do-not-resuscitate (DNR) orders
retinoblastoma, 57
rightness or wrongness. *See* ethics; principles; rights; standards
rights. *See also* ethics; principles; standards
    of father, in abortion debate, 34
    First Amendment, 193–94
    health care as public utility and/or entitlement, 266–67
    individual, emphasis on, in Western culture, 208–9
    parents with seriously ill newborns, 72

Patient Self-Determination Act, 104–5, 197
    patient's, and ADA guidelines, 141
        See also autonomy of patient
    reproductive, 33–34
rights, duties, and obligations, 12–14
risks, medicals, 118–19
Ross, W. D., 13–14

SARS, and deaths of health care providers, 179–80
Sartre, Jean-Paul, 15
Schiavo, Terri, 104, 131
sedation, terminal (or palliative), 158–59
selective abortion
    abnormalities of fetus, 40–42
    multifetal pregnancy, 2
    rape, 43–44
self-determination, 151. *See also* autonomy of patient; Patient Self-Determination Act
self-preservation, 152
sexually transmitted diseases (STDs), 169
skin integrity, patient in vegetative state, 136
sleep-wake cycles, 133
social aspects of care giving, 121–122
social services
    assistance for families with disabled children, 68
    advance directives, 103
    parens patriae, government's role as, 72–73, 195
society and abortion debate, 41
    somatic cell nuclear transfer (SCNT), 235, 237–39
"sorrow, chronic," in families with disabled children, 68
"spare" fetuses, in in vitro fertilization, 57–58
Special Committee on Biomedical Ethics, 197
spina bifida, 41–42, 73
spinal reflexes, 134
standards. *See also* ethics; principles; rights
    best interests standard, 100–1
    for treatment decision making, 69–71
    substituted judgment, 100–1, 137
    stem cell research
    case study, 234
    described, 235–36
    ethics, 236–39

stewardship of medical resources, 140
Stewart, William, 179
Stoics, the, 14
subjects, human, in medical research, 217–228
substituted judgment, standard of, 100–1, 137
suicide, assisted. *See* assisted suicide
supererogation, act of, 44
surrogacy, arguments for and against, 54–56

testing, genetic, presymptomatic, 262–64
therapeutic donor insemination (TDI), 51
Thomson, James, 238
total parenteral feeding, 114
tracheostomy, 136
Transplant and Health Policy Center, 252
transplant candidates. *See* allocation; organ donation
treatment, medical. *See also* life-sustaining treatments
   effective vs. futile, and parents' right to decide, 72, 121–22
   futility of, defining, 91–92
   life-sustaining vs. euthanasia, 73–74
   ordinary vs. extraordinary, 83–84
   reliably expected to benefit, 69
   standards, for seriously ill newborns, 69–73
   vs. standard care, 115–17
   withdrawing, vs. euthanasia, 87
truth-telling
   in communication, 19–20
   about terminal illness, 205–8, 211
tube feeding, 85
Tuskegee Syphilis Study, 218
twinning, and abortion debate, 37
twins, case study, 53–56

unconsciousness. *See also* consciousness
   advance directives, 103
   American Diabetic Association guidelines for care, 141
   criteria for diagnosing vegetative states, 133–34
   living will, 101–2
United Network for Organ Sharing (UNOS), 250–51
Urbani, Dr. Carolo, 179–80

U.S. Department of Health and Human Services
   consent, free and informed, of patients, 226
   Health Insurance Portability and Accountability Act (HIPAA), 172–73
   institutional review boards (IRBs), 218
U.S. Department of Public Health, 218
U.S. Office for Civil Rights, 6
utilitarianism
   abortion debate, 41
   assisted suicide and euthanasia, 11–12, 152
   artificial insemination debate, 52, 53
   confidentiality, 9
   consequences of actions, 10
   organ donation, 249–50
   see also Kantian ethics

Vatican Congregation for the Doctrine of the Faith, 116–17
vegetative state, patient in
   assisted nutrition and hydration, 136
   benefits and burdens, weighing, 137
   case study, 132–33
   criteria for diagnosing, 133–34
   decision making, 136–40
   disabled vs. dying, 138–40
   infections and care for, 136–38
   life expectancy, 135–36
   pain, reflex vs. conscious experience of, 135
   persistent vs. permanent, 133–36
   preventive care, 136
   terminology debated, 134–35
ventilator
   -dependent, and organ donation, 245
   palliative care, 86

waiting list exchange, for organ donation, 249, 251
weighing benefits and burdens. *See* benefits and burdens, weighing
welfare
   of children, and surrogacy, 55–56
   of incapacitated adults, 100–1
will, living. *See* living will
Willowbrook hepatitis experiments, 218

Wisconsin Cancer Pain Initiative, 158
withholding vs. withdrawing life-sustaining treatment, 86–87
women
    changing status and ethics, 18
    exploiting, for reproductive technologies and research, 54–56, 239
    rape, and abortion debate, 43–44
    reproductive rights, 33–34
World Medical Association, 218